Families and Health:
Cross-Cultural Perspectives

Families and Health: Cross-Cultural Perspectives has been co-published simultaneously as *Journal of Family Social Work*, Volume 6, Number 1 2001.

Families and Health: Cross-Cultural Perspectives

Jorge Delva, PhD
Editor

Families and Health: Cross-Cultural Perspectives has been co-published simultaneously as *Journal of Family Social Work*, Volume 6, Number 1 2001

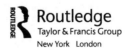

Routledge
Taylor & Francis Group
New York   London

First published by

The Haworth Social Work Practice Press®, 10 Alice Street, Binghamton, NY 13904-1580 USA

The Haworth Social Work Practice Press® is an imprint of The Haworth Press, Inc., 10 Alice Street, Binghamton, NY 13904-1580 USA.

This edition published 2012 by Routledge

Routledge
Taylor & Francis Group
711 Third Avenue
New York, NY 10017

Routledge
Taylor & Francis Group
2 Park Square, Milton Park
Abingdon, Oxon OX14 4RN

Families and Health: Cross-Cultural Perspectives has been co-published simultaneously as *Journal of Family Social Work,* Volume 6, Number 1 2001.

The development, preparation, and publication of this work has been undertaken with great care. However, the publisher, employees, editors, and agents of The Haworth Press and all imprints of The Haworth Press, Inc., including The Haworth Medical Press® and Pharmaceutical Products Press®, are not responsible for any errors contained herein or for consequences that may ensue from use of materials or information contained in this work. Opinions expressed by the author(s) are not necessarily those of The Haworth Press, Inc.

Cover design by Thomas J. Mayshock Jr.

Library of Congress Cataloging-in-Publication Data

Families and health : cross-cultural perspectives / Jorge Delva, editor.
    p. cm.
    "Co-published simultaneously as Journal of family social work volume 6, number 1 2001."
    Includes bibliographical references and index.
    ISBN 0-7890-1658-3 (hard : alk. paper)–ISBN 0-7890-1659-1 (pbk: alk. paper)
    1. Family–Health and hygiene. 2. Family–Mental health. 3. Sick–Family relationships. I. Delva, Jorge. II. Journal of family social work. V. 6, no. 1 (Supplement)
  RC455.4.F3 F3577 2001
  362.1'042–DC21   2001039739

ABOUT THE EDITOR

Jorge Delva, PhD, is Assistant Professor in the School of Social Work at Florida State University. A native of Chile, he received his doctorate in social welfare from the University of Hawaii where he learned to truly appreciate diversity and the important role that culture plays in a person's development, health and functioning. His interest in cultures led him to study Mandarin, Japanese, and some Samoan. Recently, Dr. Delva completed a two-year postdoctoral fellowship in drug epidemiology at The Johns Hopkins University funded by the National Institute on Drug Abuse. While at Hopkins, he assisted with the development of school-based drug surveys in several countries in Central America. His most recent projects involve evaluating the effectiveness of Florida's substance abuse treatment services and studying the occurrence of drug use as a multi-level phenomenon among individuals of racial and ethnic minorities using data from the National Household Survey on Drug Abuse.

Families and Health:
Cross-Cultural Perspectives

CONTENTS

A Study of Attitudes Toward Aging and Caregiving Patterns Among Samoan Families in Hawaii

Debora S. Tauiliili, MSW
Jorge Delva, PhD
Colette Browne, DrPH

SUMMARY. The purpose of this study was to examine the relationship of attitudes toward the aged and family caregiving patterns among Samoan men and women in Hawaii, taking into consideration gender and age differences. The findings revealed that both caregivers and non-caregivers held positive attitudes toward aging. Among caregivers, those with more positive attitudes toward the aged provided more personal care and chore services to an aged family member. In contrast to national studies, no gender and age differences in attitudes towards the elderly were observed among caregivers. Implications for the delivery of culturally-sensitive services to this growing Asian and Pacific Islander population are presented. *[Article copies available for a fee from The Haworth Document Delivery Service: 1-800-342-9678. E-mail address:*

Debora S. Tauiliili resides in Tallahassee, Florida. Jorge Delva is Assistant Professor, Florida State University, School of Social Work. Colette Browne is Associate Professor, University of Hawaii, School of Social Work.

Address correspondence to: Jorge Delva, PhD, Florida State University, Tallahassee, FL 32306-2570.

The authors express special appreciation to High Chief Tauiliili of American Samoa for his assistance in translation and guidance in this study. Also, the authors would like to thank Dr. Joel Fischer for his helpful comments in the preparation of the manuscript.

[Haworth co-indexing entry note]: "A Study of Attitudes Toward Aging and Caregiving Patterns Among Samoan Families in Hawaii." Tauiliili. Debora S., Jorge Delva, and Colette Browne. Co-published simultaneously in *Journal of Family Social Work* (The Haworth Social Work Practice Press, an imprint of The Haworth Press, Inc.) Vol. 6, No. 1, 2001, pp. 1-14; and: *Families and Health: Cross-Cultural Perspectives* (ed: Jorge Delva) The Haworth Social Work Practice Press, an imprint of The Haworth Press, Inc., 2001, pp. 1-14. Single or multiple copies of this article are available for a fee from The Haworth Document Delivery Service [1-800-342-9678. 9:00 a.m. - 5:00 p.m. (EST). E-mail address: getinfo@ haworthpressinc.com].

<getinfo@haworthpressinc.com> Website: <http://www.HaworthPress.com> © 2001 by The
Haworth Press, Inc. All rights reserved.]

KEYWORDS. Minority aged, caregiving, attitudes on age, Samoan elders, gender differences

Families provide the bulk of the care of the aged, with such care often defined in the literature as family caregiving. Given the rapidly increasing costs of long term care, researchers, policy makers, and practitioners have become interested in identifying those factors that influence the family's decision to provide caregiving at home (Rabiner, 1992). Recent attention to the diversity in the United States' (U.S.) population has led to increased focus on the importance of ethnicity in family caregiving and service utilization (Falcone & Broyles, 1994; Mui & Burnette, 1994).

A growing interest in gerontology is a focus on ethnic variations in caregiving of the aged. Researchers have focused on the relationships between cultural values and caregiving but have neglected to examine the relationship between ethnic variations in attitudes toward older persons and caregiving. Understanding a group's attitudes is critical because changes in attitudes are eventually reflected in a cultural group's mode of conduct (Rokeach, 1973). This study measures the relationships among attitudes toward the aged, gender, and age upon family caregiving patterns among an adult Samoan population in Hawaii. Cultural variations in caregiving and caregiving patterns in the United States are reviewed.

BACKGROUND ON THE RESEARCH POPULATION

The United States recently has become the major destination for Pacific migration from the Samoas, Tonga, and Fiji (Barker, 1990). According to the 1990 Census report, Samoans number more than 60,000 and are the second largest Polynesian population in the United States, surpassed only by Hawaiians (U.S. Census Bureau, 1993). Hawaii and California are the favored destinations for Samoans who have immigrated from Samoa, and more often than not they reside in the major cities of these states (Barker, 1990).

A number of reasons have been given for the high rate of migration–the economic changes in American Samoa, the desire to join families already in the U.S., and the relative ease to migrate to the U.S. (Browne & Broderick, 1991; Franco, 1987). Literature on Samoans in the United States is sparse and exact data on service utilization is unknown. This lack of data, along with limited knowledge on the attitudes, cultural practices, and behaviors of Samoans in the United States, has impeded the design and delivery of culturally-relevant services.

Attitudes Toward the Aged in the United States and Samoa

Austin (1985) notes that the social role of members of any cultural group depend on social attitudes others hold toward them. Hooyman and Kiyak (1993) reviewed the literature on attitudes toward aging and found that the majority of Americans hold either neutral or positive attitudes toward aging. Researchers interested in the dynamics of culture have hypothesized that certain cultural values found among Asian and Pacific cultures, such as filial piety and familism, are more often associated with societies that revere their aged (Braun et al., 1995).

In contrast to American values that stress independence and individuality, Samoan cultural values emphasize cooperation and interdependence, communal relations, and the key roles of the family and the church (Mokuau & Chang, 1991). Historically, Samoans look favorably to growing old for old age represents a time when a person can relax and have other family members look after them (Holmes, 1983). While such observations point to positive attitudes about aging in general, specific attitudes toward the aged have not been formally measured. The measure of such attitudes by Samoans in the United States is important because studies indicate that Samoan immigrants are encouraged to assimilate by becoming more individualistic and assertive (Pearson, 1992). The adoption of Western values may affect Samoan attitudes toward the aged, and the Samoan family's caregiving patterns of their aged.

Cultural Variations in Caregiving

Increasing evidence points to ethnic variations in caregiving and service use in the U.S. (Luborshy & Sankar, 1993; Mui & Burnette, 1994) and across nations (Choi, 1993; Sung, 1990). Studies on cross cultural caregiving have recently focused on describing culturally-linked values as a positive influence on caregiving patterns (Henrichsen & Ramirez,

1992). Other studies have examined ethnic variations in caregiving and service use and suggest that structural barriers such as economic status and discriminatory service practices account for ethnic differences in service use and care patterns (Falcone & Broyles, 1994). Still other studies have examined ethnic variations in caregiving among pre-industrial or rural societies and have either supported or refuted the modernization theory (Glascock, 1990; Quadagno, 1982). Briefly, this theory states that there is an inverse relationship between the degree a society has become modernized and its attitudes toward the aged (Cowgill, 1986). Pearson's (1992) study provided some support to this theory. He investigated the influences of modernization toward elderly Samoans in rural Samoa (formerly known as Western Samoa, an independent country and the least Americanized), American Samoa (Americanized), and urban Honolulu (the most Americanized). Whereas the aged were respected and obeyed in all three sites, Samoans in American Samoa and Honolulu reported declines in the elderly Samoan's status over the past ten years.

Changes in attitudes may impact the care of aged Samoans. For example, *fa'a Samoa* or the Samoan Way of Life, has underscored home care for its aged and resulted in policy makers and planners placing more emphasis on home and community services than on nursing home care (Browne & Broderick, 1991). Whether or not changes in attitudes on aging impact caregiving patterns and the use of services is important data that need to be collected to develop a culturally-responsive service-delivery system of care.

Gender, Age, and Caregiving Patterns in the United States

Families are the majority of the caregivers of the frail aged in the U.S., and caregiving has become a critical personal and public policy issue. Several studies have identified the primary caregiver as most often the spouse, a wife, or an adult child, usually a daughter or daughter-in-law (Anastas, Gibeau, & Larson, 1990; Stone, Cafferata, & Sangl, 1986). Indeed, gender and age have a strong relationship to the provision of caregiving. Middle-aged women comprise over 75 percent of family caregivers to the aged who are chronically ill (Tennstedt, McKinlay, & Sullivan, 1989). Women's caregiving role has generally been attributed to cultural and socialization processes that define women as nurturers of the young, the aged, and the infirm. In response to this national caregiver profile, social work programs have typically targeted the middle aged woman for services, and the services most often provided are support groups, education on community services, and stress reduction services (Barnes, Given, & Given, 1995; Hooyman & Kiyak, 1993). However, information on caregiving patterns and attitudes towards the elderly among different ethnocultural groups is clearly lacking (Braun et al., 1995). In view of this deficiency, the present study seeks to study the association between attitudes towards the elderly and caregiving patterns among Samoan families in Hawaii. In addition, gender differences and age differences in attitudes and care are explored.

METHOD

Four hypotheses guided this study of Samoan families' caregiving practices in Hawaii. These hypotheses were formulated as follows: (a) Individual caregivers who provide care to an older relative (55 and above) will differ on their attitudes toward the aged compared to individual noncaregivers (those who do not provide care to an older relative); (b) among caregivers, there will be a relationship between attitudes towards the aged and caregiving patterns; (c) there are gender differences in caregiving patterns of Samoan families in Hawaii; and (d) there is a relationship between the age of the caregiver and caregiving patterns. In this study, caregiver was defined as a respondent who has an older Samoan relative (age 55+) living in the same household. Caregiving patterns were defined by whether personal care and chore services were provided by Samoans in Hawaii to elder Samoans living in the same household. Personal care was defined as bathing, dressing, feeding, and giving of medications to the older relative living in the household. Chore services were defined as activities the caregiver provided for the older adult and included food preparation, housecleaning, laundry and shopping.

Sample

Participants in the study were a purposive sample of 85 adult Samoans (over 18 years of age) recruited from four local churches on Oahu, the most populous island of Hawaii. These four Samoan congregations were selected for the study because they are among the most widely attended Samoan churches in Honolulu. Studies have shown that 99% of the Samoan population in Samoa claim membership in a church (Holmes, 1983).

6 FAMILIES AND HEALTH: CROSS-CULTURAL PERSPECTIVES

Procedures

An introductory letter was sent to pastors of each church, briefly stating the purpose of the study and seeking the agreement of the pastor to conduct the study. Following their agreement, procedures were made for the pastors to distribute the questionnaire to the church members (i.e., after church services). The questionnaire included a cover letter describing the study, a consent form to participate in the study, and the questionnaire. Fifty questionnaires were distributed by the pastors of each congregation to participants during church gatherings, for a total of 200 questionnaires. They were instructed by the pastors to return them by the following week. The total response rate was 85 or 43%.

Instruments

A self-administered questionnaire was used for this study and consisted of three sections. The first section asked participants to describe their caregiving patterns of the aged. The second section examined attitudes towards the aged. The third section sought sociodemographic information of respondents. The questionnaire was provided in both Samoan and English. The questionnaire was translated and checked by a Samoan individual who holds the ranks of "High Chief" and "Talking Chief" in the Samoan Islands. Revisions to the instrument were made accordingly. Also, the instrument was pilot tested for comprehensibility and length with three Samoan native speakers in Hawaii. It took these individuals an average of 15 minutes to complete the questionnaire.

Caregiving Status and Patterns. To determine if one was a caregiver we asked the following question: Does an older relative (those who are 55 years and older) live with you? Older relative was defined as being 55 years or older because this particular age (55) is an indicator of developmental changes (e.g., changes in roles and responsibilities) of the Samoan people (Holmes & Rhoads, 1983; Rhoads, 1984). To determine caregiving patterns, two questions were asked which required a "YES" or "NO" response. Face validity was attained through discussions with professionals in gerontology settings in Hawaii and discussions by Samoan community experts in both American Samoa and Hawaii. The two questions are:

- Some older adults need help with their bathing, dressing, feeding, and giving of medications. Do you provide this kinds of care to this older relative(s)?

• Other older adults may need help with food preparation, housecleaning, laundry and shopping. Do you provide these kinds of
chore services to this older relative(s)?

Attitudes Toward the Aged. Kite and Johnson (1988) reviewed several
instruments used to measure attitude towards aging and concluded that no
instrument was best to measure this construct. Of the various instruments
to measure attitudes toward the aged, Tuckman and Lorge's (1953) was selected for this study. The primary criteria for the selection of this instrument was that its intent is to evaluate attitudes; other instruments tend to
assess constructs not needed for this study such as knowledge, intentions,
or preferences. This instrument has 137 statements which asks the respondent to respond with a "YES" (score = 1) if they agree or "NO" (score = 0)
if they disagree with the statement. Scores range from 1 to 137, with lower
scores indicating more positive attitudes toward the aged. An example of a
statement is: They (older adults) should not marry . . . Yes/No. Scoring of
the instrument allows for a total score that measures attitude towards the
aged. The psychometric properties have been found to be adequate. Specifically, test-retest reliability coefficients have ranged from .36 to .62 depending on whether the responses apply to middle age or to older
individuals, the later having higher coefficients (Axelford & Eisdorfer,
1961). Two studies of college students' attitudes towards the elderly found
statistically significant differences in attitudes towards 35-, 45-, 55-, 65-,
and 75-year-old individuals, with the older groups receiving a higher number of stereotypic responses (Axelford & Eisdorfer, 1961; Eisdorfer, 1966).
These findings suggest adequate criterion-related validity.

RESULTS

Characteristics of the Respondents

Among this sample, 37 or 43.5% were caregivers and 48 or 56.5%
were noncaregivers. The ratio of males and females in both groups was
very similar. Among caregivers, there were 19 (51%) females and 18
(49%) males. In the noncaregiver group, there were 21 (46%) females
and 25 (54%) males, with two respondents who did not identify their
gender (see Table 1). Educationally, caregivers had less education than
noncaregivers but these differences were not statistically significant,
$(\chi^2(4, N = 83) = 2.98, p > .05)$. Income differences between caregivers

TABLE 1. Demographic Characteristics of Caregivers and Noncaregivers

Demographic	Caregiver		Noncaregiver	
	n	%	n	%
Total	37	100	48	100
Age	34	100	43	100
20-29	13	38.0	13	30.0
30-39	7	21.0	12	28.0
40-49	8	23.0	10	23.0
50-54	6	18.0	8	19.0
Sex	37	100	46	100
Female	19	51.4	21	45.7
Male	18	48.6	25	54.3
Marital Status	37	100	48	100
Never Married	8	21.6	8	15.0
Married	21	56.8	37	79.0
Divorced	4	10.8	0	0
Widowed	4	10.8	3	6.0
Education Level	37	100	46	100
Elementary	3	8.0	1	2.2
High School	18	49.0	27	58.7
Church School	5	14.0	3	6.5
College	9	24.0	13	28.3
No Formal Education	2	5.0	2	4.3
Family's Annual Income in ($)	34	100	46	100
5,000-14,999	14	41.0	23	50.0
15,000-24,999	6	18.0	9	19.0
25,000-34,999	1	3.0	5	11.0
35,000 or more	4	12.0	6	13.0
Don't Know	9	26.0	3	7.0

Note. Not all respondents answered all the demographic questions. Thus, in some categories, the total number of respondents is less than the total number of caregivers (N = 37) and noncaregivers (N = 48).

and noncaregivers were not statistically significant ($\chi^2(19, N = 80) = 18.07, p > .05$, with caregivers earning slightly more than noncaregivers.

Nearly three-fourths of caregivers and two-third of noncaregivers have lived in Hawaii for more than 11 years. In spite of the migration to the United States, the Samoan language remains as the primary language spoken at home by individuals in both caregiving (90%) and noncaregiving (80%) groups. In sum, an analysis of the demographic information indicates that both groups are quite similar in their sociodemographic characteristics.

Hypotheses Tested

The first hypothesis tested was that there was no difference in attitudes toward the aged between caregivers and noncaregivers. An independent t-test indicated that the difference in attitude scores between caregivers (M = 81.7) and noncaregivers (M = 87.3) was not statistically significant, $(t(83) = .11, p > .05)$. Similarly, the differences in attitude scores between caregivers and noncaregivers by gender and age of the respondents were not statistically significant (see Table 2). Thus, Samoan men and women, old and young, in both groups share similar positive attitudes towards the elderly.

The second hypothesis examined whether there was a relationship between attitudes towards the aged and caregiving patterns among caregivers (defined as individuals who provide personal care and chore services). Among caregivers, there was a significant correlation between positive attitude towards the aged and those who provided personal care, $(r(37) = .41, p < .05)$ and chore services $(r(36) = .45, p < .01)$. In other words, caregivers who provided personal care and chore services had more positive attitudes towards aging than caregivers who did not provide personal care or chore services.

The third hypothesis tested whether there were gender differences in caregiving patterns of Samoan families in Hawaii. Results from a chi-square analysis indicated that the number of males and females that provided personal care and chore services did not differ significantly (see Table 3).

The fourth hypothesis examined whether the caregiving patterns of caregivers differed as a function of the caregivers' age. Two age groups were formed, 20-29 and 30-54. These groups were selected to be consistent with the age breakdown of Tuckman and Lorge's (1953) analysis for comparison purposes. Results indicated that individuals in the 20-29 age group are as likely as individuals in the 30-54 age group to provide personal care $(\chi^2(1, n = 34) = 1.4, p > .05)$ and chore services $(\chi^2(1, n = 33 = 1.42, p > .05)$. These data show that care for an aged relative is distributed equally between younger and older individuals.

DISCUSSION

This study examined the attitudes toward aging and caregiving patterns among a sample of Samoan families residing in Hawaii. Overall,

TABLE 2. Mean Scores of Variable Attitude Toward the Aged by Group, Gender and Age

	Caregiver			Noncaregiver		
	n	M	sd	n	M	sd
Total	37	81.7	28.6	48	87.3	30.0*
Gender						
Female	19	87.9	29.2	21	89.1	21.2
Male	18	76.2	26.5	25	86.4	36.0
Age Group						
20-29	13	78.0	28.5	13	89.5	39.7
30-54	21	84.4	30.3	30	84.1	23.1

Note. The sample size for the gender and age categories does not add to the total number of respondents (N = 85) as two respondents did not indicate their gender and eight did not indicate their age.
*$p < .05$.

TABLE 3. Number of Caregivers Who Provide Personal Care and Chore Services by Gender

	Personal Care		Chore Services	
	Yes	No	Yes	No
Female	11	8	17	2
Male	10	8	14	3

$\chi^2(1, n = 37) = 1.39, p > .05$
$\chi^2(1, n = 36) = 1.38, p > .05$

there were no statistically significant differences in positive attitudes toward aging among caregivers compared to noncaregivers. Such data provide support to previous studies that describe most Samoans as having positive attitudes toward older persons (Cowgill, 1986; Holmes & Rhoads, 1983). On the other hand, the data suggest that caregivers who provided more personal care and chore services tend to have more positive attitudes toward aging than did the caregivers who provided less personal care or chore services to an older relative. This finding suggests a number of different explanations. A first explanation is that positive attitudes may well influence the decision to provide personal care or chore services or the amount of such care to an older relative. In other words, more positive attitudes may result in a greater willingness to provide personal or chore help. However, it may also be that the provision of more services at home results in more positive attitudes toward the aged if one's culture respects the aged and if the family's prestige in the Samoan community is elevated by the provision of such care. Such an explanation receives some support in the literature. For example, in their discussion of family care patterns and roles, Mokuau and Chang (1991) state that "the members of the Samoan family experience a true sense of communal relationship because there is a sharing of roles and responsibilities" (p. 160). In other words, providing eldercare may place the family in such a positive light in their own community that positive attitudes develop toward the care recipient.

The third and fourth hypotheses investigated the relationships between gender and age to caregiving respectively. Contrary to national profiles of American caregivers, there were no significant difference in caregiving patterns by gender or by age. A gender division of labor does exist among Samoans but apparently not in the care of the aged, at least in this sample. In traditional and contemporary Samoan culture, men are the providers and women are the caretakers of the young. The results of this study suggest that responsibility for the care of an older Samoan relative is provided regardless of the gender or age of the caregiver. These data support other studies in noting ethnic variations in caregiving patterns (Mui & Burnette, 1994), but do not support others (Stone, Cafferata, & Sangl, 1986) that describe caregivers as primarily women and middle aged. Clearly, such data argue against overgeneralizations and stereotypes about Samoan caregivers and their needs.

These findings are subject to a number of limitations. We had defined caregivers as those families who provided care to an elder in their own home. Using this definition, noncaregivers could in fact be providing care to an older adult not in the same household, a question not asked in this study. Data limitations could also be due to immigration patterns, with many Samoan elder relatives still in American or Western Samoa. Families often provide remittances, payment to their elders in Samoa, but such behavior would not have constituted caregiving behaviors as defined by this study. Furthermore, and despite increasing conceptual work in the area of cultural variations in caregiving, there is at present no direct measure of culturally-linked attitudes or behaviors that could assist us in this study. Another caveat of this study is the lack of conceptual clarity between attitudes toward aging and values (Webber, Coombs & Hollingsworth, 1974) and the lack of a standardized instrument on attitudes on aging (Kite & Johnson, 1988). The Tuckman and Lorge (1953) measurement tool to assess attitudes on aging, while adequate, may not have been culturally sensitive to pick up statements that were applicable to the Samoan culture. Finally, as a cross sectional study, this study could not measure the potential impact of acculturation over time on changing attitudes on aging and family caregiving patterns. Nonetheless, this study is unique in measuring intraethnic variations among Samoans in the caregiving of their aged, and suggests a number of implications for social work.

Implications for Social Work Practice

These results suggest that Samoans in our sample do hold positive attitudes toward the aged. Also, the results also suggest that those with more positive attitudes provide more personal care and chore services to an older relative compared to those with less positive attitudes. As there were no differences in gender and age of caregivers in caregiving patterns, these data suggest that interventions be designed and conducted to include all members of the family rather than target only women as many programs have done. Social workers should not be surprised when all members of the immediate and extended family are present in a family meeting. Finally, while Samoan families appear to have positive attitudes toward the aged, the combination of insensitive programs and economic hardships may make the job of caring for the aged a difficult and challenging one. The provision of culturally competent services and interventions to benefit all caregivers and older adults requires a commitment to understanding and responding both to a diverse aging population and those who care for them.

REFERENCES

Anastas, J., Gibeau, J.L., & Larson, P.J. (1990). Working families and eldercare: A National perspective in an aging America. *Social Work, 35,* 405-411.

Austin, D. (1985). Attitudes toward old age: A hierarchical study. *Gerontologist, 25,* 431-434.

Axelrod, S., & Eisdorfer, C. (1961). Attitudes toward older people: An Empirical analysis of the stimulus group validity of the Tuckman Lorge Questionnaire. *Journal of Gerontology, 16,* 75-80.

Barker, J. (1990). Pacific Island migrants in the United States: Some implications for aging services. *Journal of Cross Cultural Gerontology, 6,* 173-192.

Barnes, C.L., Given, B.A., & Given, C.W. (1995). Patient caregivers: A Comparison of employed and not employed daughters. *Social Work, 40,* 375-381.

Braun, K., Takamura, J., Forman, S., Sasaki, P., & Meinenger, L. (1995). Developing and testing outreach materials on Alzheimer's Disease for Asian and Pacific Islander Americans. *Gerontologist, 35,* 122-126.

Browne, C., & Broderick, A. (1991). *Aging and ethnicity: A replication handbook for social work education for practice with Asian and Pacific Island elders.* Honolulu: University of Hawaii

Choi, H. (1993). Cultural and noncultural factors as determinants of caregiver burden for the impaired elderly in South Korea. *Gerontologist, 33,* 8-15.

Cowgill, D. (1986). *Aging around the world.* Belmont, CA: Wadsworth.

Eisdorfer, C. (1966). Attitudes toward old people: A re-analysis of the item validity of the stereotype scale. *Journal of Gerontology, 21,* 455-462.

Falcone, D., & Broyles, R. (1994). Access to long term care: Race is a barrier. *Journal of Health, Politics, Policy, and Law, 19,* 583-595.

Franco, R. W. (1987). *Samoans in Hawaii: A sociodemographic profile.* Honolulu, HI: East West Center.

Glascock, A. P. (1990). By any other name, it is still killing: A Comparison of the treatment of the elderly in American and other societies. In J. Sokolovsky (Ed.), *The Cultural context of aging: World perspectives* (pp. 43-56). New York: Bergen and Gary.

Henrichsen, G., & Ramirez, M. (1992). Black and white dementia caregivers: A comparison of their adaptation, adjustment, and service utilization. *Gerontologist, 33,* 375-381.

Holmes, L. (1983). *Other cultures, elder years: An introduction to cultural gerontology.* Minneapolis, MN: Burgess.

Holmes, L., & Rhoads, E. (1983). Aging and change in Samoa: In J. Sokolovsky (Ed.), *Growing old in different societies* (3y rd ed.). Belmont, CA: Wadsworth.

Hooyman, N., & Kiyak, H. (1993) (3rd edition). *Social gerontology: A multidisciplinary perspective* (3rd ed.). Needham Heights: Allyn and Bacon.

Kite, M.E., & Johnson, B.T. (1988). Attitudes toward older and young adults: A meta-analysis. *Psychology and Aging, 2,* 233-244.

Luborshy, M., & Sankar, A. (1993). Extending the critical gerontology perspective: Cultural dimensions. *Gerontologist, 33,* 440-444.

Mokuau, N., & Chang, N. (1991). Samoans. In N. Mokuau (Ed.), *Handbook of social services for Asian and Pacific Islanders* (pp. 155-169). Westport, CT: Greenwood.

Mui, A.C., & Burnette, D. (1994). Long term care service use by frail elders: Is ethnicity a factor? *Gerontologist, 34,* 190-198.

Pearson, J. D. (1992). Attitudes and perceptions concerning elderly Samoans in rural Western Samoa, American Samoa, and urban Honolulu. *Journal of Cross-Cultural Gerontology, 7,* 69-88.

Quadagno, J. (1982). *Aging in early industrial society.* New York: Academic Press.

Rabiner, D.J. (1992). The relationship between program participation, use of formal in-home care, and satisfaction with care in an elderly population. *Gerontologist, 32,* 805-812.

Rhoads, E. (1984). The Impact of modernization on the aged in American Samoa. *Pacific Studies, 7,* 15-33.

Rokeach, M. (1973). *The Nature of human values.* New York: Free Press.

Stone, R., Cafferata, G., & Sangl, S. (1986). *Caregivers of the frail: A national profile.* Washington D.C., U.S. Department of Labor.

Sung, K. (1990). A new look at filial piety: Ideals and practices of family centered parent care in Korea. *Gerontologist, 30,* 610-617.

Tennstedt, S.L., Crawford, S., & McKinley, J.B. (1993). Is family care on the decline? A Longitudinal investigation of the substitute of formal long term care services with informal care. *Millbank Quarterly, 7,* 620-624.

Tuckman, J., & Lorge, I. (1953). Attitudes toward old people. *Journal of Social Psychology, 37,* 249-260.

United States Bureau of the Census. (1993). *Asian and Pacific Islanders in the United States by ethnicity.* Summary Tape File 1C. Washington, DC: Bureau of the Census.

Webber, I.W., Coombs, D.W., & Hollingworth, J.S. (1974). Variations in value orientations by age in a developing society. *Journal of Gerontology, 29,* 676-683.

Searching for Family:
Voices of Florida's Foster Children

Sally G. Mathiesen, PhD
Brenda "BJ" Jarmon, PhD
Leslie Clarke, PhD

SUMMARY. The growing shortage of foster homes in Florida and new challenges to recruiting foster parents prompted the Florida Department of Children and Families (DCF) to commission a statewide study. The study was designed to identify the perceptions of foster parents, foster children, Department staff and other agency representatives concerning ways to improve foster parent recruitment and retention.

This paper presents the purpose and scope of the study, and the state of foster care in the United States (U.S.) and Florida. In particular, we focus on the perceptions of the foster teens in the sample and their ideas to improve foster parent recruitment and retention, as well as methodological challenges to interviewing foster parents and children. A consistent theme noted by the teenagers was that they thought some parents were dedicated to giving a good home and support to children in need. Foster children also reported that monetary concerns played a major role in people choosing to foster or remaining in foster parenting. Many children

---

Sally G. Mathiesen is affiliated with the Florida State University, School of Social Work. Brenda "BJ" Jarmon is affiliated with the Florida Agricultural and Mechanical University. Leslie Clarke is affiliated with the University of Florida.

The authors gratefully acknowledge the support received for this research through a grant from the State of Florida Department of Children and Families via the Lawton and Rhea Chiles Center for Healthy Mothers and Babies.

[Haworth co-indexing entry note]: "Searching for Family: Voices of Florida's Foster Children." Mathiesen, Sally G., Brenda "BJ" Jarmon, and Leslie Clarke. Co-published simultaneously in *Journal of Family Social Work* (The Haworth Social Work Practice Press, an imprint of The Haworth Press, Inc.) Vol. 6, No. 1, 2001, pp. 15-33; and: *Families and Health: Cross-Cultural Perspectives* (ed: Jorge Delva) The Haworth Social Work Practice Press, an imprint of The Haworth Press, Inc., 2001, pp. 15-33. Single or multiple copies of this article are available for a fee from The Haworth Document Delivery Service [1-800-342-9678, 9:00 a.m. - 5:00 p.m. (EST). E-mail address: getinfo@haworthpressinc.com].

15

are in foster care many years longer than they should be and often experience multiple foster homes, making if difficult for them to feel secure. Specific attention is given to the implications for family social work practice. *[Article copies available for a fee from The Haworth Document Delivery Service: 1-800-342-9678. E-mail address: <getinfo@haworthpressinc.com> Website: <http://www.HaworthPress.com> © 2001 by The Haworth Press, Inc. All rights reserved.]*

KEYWORDS. Foster care, children, and youths evaluation

INTRODUCTION

The growing shortage of foster homes in Florida and new challenges to recruiting foster parents prompted the Florida Department of Children and Families (DCF) to commission a statewide study. The study was designed to identify the perceptions of foster parents, foster children, Department staff and other agency representatives concerning ways to improve foster parent recruitment and retention.

The goals of this study were:

- to provide information to the Florida Department of Children and Families (DCF) on current activities and trends in foster care recruitment and retention;
- to identify the perceptions of foster parents, foster children, Department staff and other agency representatives concerning ways to improve foster parent recruitment and retention; and
- to develop a plan for improving recruitment and retention of foster parents.

The study was commissioned because of the growing demand for foster homes and the increasing difficulty the Department has experienced in recruiting and keeping foster families. This paper focuses on the "voices" of the foster children, one of the stakeholder groups addressed in the larger study. The perceptions of the foster children in the study regarding recruitment and retention of foster parents are presented and the potential impact for family social work practice is discussed.

National Trends in Foster Care

The foster care population in the United States has increased dramatically in the past decade. As reported by the Administration for

Children, Youth and Families (2000), there were more than 500,000 children in foster care in 1996, and 280,000 in care in 1986. The Child Welfare League of America (2000) reported that sixty percent of children in care in 1998 returned to their birth families, after spending an average of 33 months in foster care.

In 1989, reports from the U.S. General Accounting Office (U.S. GAO) cited the lack of foster homes as a serious problem:

> Nearly every state is experiencing a serious shortage of foster families. In some states the shortage is so great the children are being shuttled from one place to another, such as temporary homes, institutions, hospitals, until a proper home is found. There are reports that children, even preschool children, are being placed in childcare institutions because appropriate foster homes are not available. Some children are sent to shelters or back to their birth home where problems may get worse. (p. 13)

Hernandez (1993) identified a number of reasons for this shortage, including the growth of two income families, the reduction of income for working families in lower socioeconomic levels, an increased number of children in out-of-home care, and high levels of separation and divorce. In addition, the U.S.GAO (1989) concluded that recruitment was also affected by the fact that reimbursement for foster care services was too low to cover all the costs of the foster child.

Characteristics of Foster Children

The age distribution of foster children in the U.S. is changing. The largest group of children in March 1998 was in the 6-10 year old range (28%), though children and teenagers from ages 11-15 (27%) and 16-18 (13%) constitute a large proportion of foster children, many of whom will age out of the system rather than become adopted (Administration for Children, Youth and Families, 2000).

The racial/ethnic distribution of children in foster care has also been changing in recent years and does not reflect the distribution of population groups in the United States. Babb (1999) reported that African American children represent 15 percent of the U.S. child population, but they represent 40 percent of all foster children who are free for adoption. The disparity in the distribution of the foster care population as compared to the U.S. population as a whole has profound implications for the recruitment of foster parents who have the same race/ethnic and cultural backgrounds as the children who need placement. The majority of foster families in the U.S. are Caucasian and the proportion of African American foster families has declined in recent years.

Emotional and Behavioral Problems of Foster Children

In a study by McIntyre and Keesler (1986) the authors found that half of foster care children "manifest evidence of psychological disorder" (p. 302), a finding "that has been widely corroborated in a variety of studies" (Epstein, 1999, p. 55). Klee and Halfon's study (1987) found that despite the great need for mental health services for foster children, their needs are routinely ignored. Fanshel, Finch, and Grundy (1989) reported that children who have experienced multiple placements display greater behavioral problems than those with single placements. In 1998, children in care in the U.S. had an average of 3.2 different foster care placements (U.S. Department of Health and Human Services, 1999). Berrick, Courtney, and Barth (1993) found that many children in group homes in California demonstrated "acting out, aggression, sexual promiscuity, and substance abuse" (p. 461).

Other studies have found that foster children, as compared to the general population, "continue to demonstrate evidence of inadequate health supervision" (Schor, 1982, p. 526), and "are more likely to be poor and in poor health (American Academy of Pediatrics, 1994, p. 2). Foster parents cannot financially meet all of the needs of these children. In 1994, foster parents received on average $407 per month for boarding, an amount too low to support adequate care (Epstein, 1999). In addition, Zuravin, Benedict, and Somerfield (1997) note that many of those who do foster may lack the skills and motivation to be able to provide nurturing relationships, with maltreatment occurring in 25 percent of foster homes. These characteristics point to serious challenges to the system in recruiting and retaining foster parents.

Florida Trends in Foster Care

In 1989, the State of Florida's Auditor General documented the extent of the problems faced by foster children in Florida (State of Florida Department of Health and Rehabilitative Services, 1989). Through a study of case records from 1982 and 1988, this report showed that rates of delinquency, emotional disturbance and developmental disabilities among foster children had more than doubled between 1982 and 1988. Sixty-four percent of their sample had at least one behavioral problem or developmental disability and nearly one-tenth of their sample habitually used drugs or alcohol. Moreover, the report found that these children were not being properly matched with foster families who have the skills to work with these children. They further noted that although foster parents are reticent or ill prepared to serve children with developmental, medical and behavioral problems, these children comprised the majority of the foster care population.

STUDY METHODS

We designed and carried out a statewide qualitative survey of foster care recruitment and retention by interviewing "stakeholders" in the foster care system through focus groups and individual interviews. We designed this portion of the study to gather representative data from all Department of Children and Family (DCF) districts in the state. The Florida Department of Children and Families provided data on the foster child caseload, licensed foster homes, capacity of foster homes and the average length of stay of various categories of foster children.

Sampling

We selected one county in each district to represent one of three types of geographic areas in the state: rural, suburban or urban. All districts were asked to submit in electronic form a list of: (a) all current foster children in the county sampled between the ages of 13 and 18 who had been in the foster care at least six months; and (b) all foster parents/foster homes in the county sampled that had a foster care placement of at least six months and were either currently active or had been active within the past five years. We also asked for data on the race/ethnicity of foster children and foster parents to be included, along with the address and phone number of all foster homes and children. Because each district stores foster care data in slightly different ways, the form of the data submitted for this study ranged from electronic records from the Interim Child Welfare Services Information System (ICWSIS) to paper reports.

With the list of target counties, we then sampled from these counties based on the characteristics of the foster parents and children. Random samples of foster children and foster homes were selected using a random number generator. Approximately 18 foster children's names and 15 foster parent names were selected from each county for recruitment into the study. Randomly selected replacement names were provided if more names were needed to assure that at least five to ten participants would attend a focus group. We also targeted one county for the collection of data from only African American participants (Pinellas) and three for the collection of data from Hispanic participants (Pinellas, Hillsborough and Dade). Targeting and segregation in focus groups and interviews were implemented to assure that minority foster parents and children would be given a safe environment within which they could express their perceptions and experiences in foster care. Race-heterogeneous groups do not always offer this comfort for minority groups members.

Interviews

Once the samples were drawn, research teams in each region sent letters to foster parents and followed these letters with phone contacts requesting the participation of foster children or parents in focus groups in the region. Agency staff was contacted directly. Once participation was assured, focus groups and interviews were held in each region in a convenient and, often, neutral location, such as a library. Prior to the start of the groups, informed consent was obtained from all participants.

Focus groups with foster parents and children, individual interviews with DCF staff and service providers, as well as group interviews with advocacy groups were conducted in the selected counties that represented all 15 districts in Florida. Group meetings and/or focus groups were held with local foster parent associations, and Youth Advisory Board members (or Department supervisors). We also conducted individual interviews with representatives of One Church, One Child programs, Guardian Ad Litem programs and other private agencies providing foster care related services. In all, a total of 4 or more focus groups and interviews were held in each district in the state for a total of more than 105 focus groups and interviews.

The focus groups were tape-recorded and often were summarized immediately following the group discussion. We tape-recorded, summarized and analyzed these data to extract the key points and recommendations from all stakeholders. Individual interviews with respondents were also tape-recorded and documented in a similar manner.

In addition to the focus group and interview data, a written survey instrument was created based on the questions developed for the focus groups. The intent of this format was to reach individuals who were not selected for the focus groups or individual interviews, but wanted to have input. The instrument was distributed broadly across the state to foster parent associations, agency staff and other groups, who were encouraged to make additional copies and distribute as needed. More than 70 written responses were received.

After the data collection procedures and analyses were complete, a draft Executive Summary of the report was distributed to all Districts. A two-hour teleconference was held that permitted interested parties at their respective District office to participate in a "live" roundtable discussion of the findings. All Districts were represented in the teleconference, and participants consisted of District staff, foster parents, foster adolescents, and representatives from foster care agencies. There was general agreement as to the issues that emerged, and some participants offered useful enhancements that were integrated into our findings and strategies.

The biggest challenges to this study were obtaining the population of foster children and foster homes that met our criteria, and getting biological parent consents for foster children to participate in the study. The Department of Children and Families does not maintain a statewide computer system with detailed demographics on the foster children or foster homes in the State. Reports are provided by the Districts to the State office on a regular basis and these reports are compiled to report on foster children and homes, but a census of the population of children and homes is not available in a centralized location. This fact made it difficult to obtain the lists we needed for our sampling. We were required to work with each regional data coordinator and study liaison to obtain regional and county-level information on current children in placement and licensed homes that had been in the system for 6 months or more.

Once we had the samples, it was challenging to obtain consent of the biological parents to talk with the foster children. While this consent is not legally mandated, legal council with the Department of Children and Families recommended it. Local Department of Children and Families staff were asked to assist with contacting biological parents and obtaining consents for the foster children sampled for the study. This was a burden to the already over-burdened counselors, and resulted in significant delays in identifying foster children to interview. In most cases, workers were unable to find or contact the biological parents. In some counties, we were simply not able to obtain consent from enough biological parents to have a foster children's focus group. In all counties we were forced to focus on the children who were available for adoption (i.e., parental rights were terminated) because biological parent consent was not required for these children.

These challenges to our data collection highlight critical barriers in the analysis of the needs of foster children. If statewide data are not available on the characteristics and needs of the foster children, or the skills of the foster parents, then targeted recruitment and appropriate matching cannot happen. Moreover, not having access to biological parents suggests a weak link in the system between the Department and the children they serve, and the homes from which these children were removed.

With respect to the foster children, there is some possible bias in these groups. Good data on how these children may differ from children whose parents have not had their rights terminated are not available. We assume, however, that the children whose parents have had their rights terminated have been in the foster care system for a longer period of time. We also hypothesized that these children may be in foster homes that are more supportive, as foster parents were required to consent in writing to the foster child participating in the study and they had to drive the child to attend the meeting. Yet, these expectations cannot be confirmed. Due to the small sample size, the findings must be considered with caution. Research efforts to gather data from case records throughout the state regarding foster child and parent characteristics will be important to complement these pilot data, and are currently in development.

Table 1 is a summary of the focus groups and interviews that were completed in each District. The numbers represent the number of people in each group or interview. The codes associated with some of the interviews indicate whether the groups were race-specific (i.e., AA = African American only, or H = Hispanic only).

RESULTS

Number of Foster Children

Our examination of Florida trend data began with an analysis of five to ten years (1989-1999) of data on foster care. The total foster care caseload–or the number of children in foster care–was only available for five years. These data are reported in Figure 1. The total foster care caseload dropped slightly between 1995 and 1996, and then was relatively consistent through 1996 and 1997. Following 1997, a dramatic increase in the number of foster children in care occurred. Between 1997 and 1999, the total caseload increased from 15,035 to 17,255. This represents an increase of nearly 15 percent, compared to the decline in

TABLE 1. Number of Participants in Focus Groups, Group Interviews and Individual Interviews

District	County Sampled	Foster Parents Focus Groups/Group Interviews		Foster Children Focus Groups /Group Interviews		DCF Staff Interviews	Guardian Ad Litem Interviews	One Church, One Child Interviews	Private Provider Community Based Care
		Random Sample	Foster Parent Assoc. Meeting	Random Sample	Youth Advisory Board				
1	Escambia	1	1	--	1 Supervisor	1	1	1	1 CHS
2	Gadsden	14	NA	3	*	1	1	*	NA
3	Alachua	5	18	*	1	2	Refused	--	1
4	Duval	3	5	3	1	2	1	1	1 CHS
5	Pinellas	7 AA	14 AA	3 AA	--	2	--	1	--
6	Hills-Borough	3	5 H	1	1	2	--	1	1
7	Orange	13	13	11	1	1	*	1	2 CHS
8	Hendry	4	NA	2	NA	2	NA	NA	NA
9	Palm Beach	11	1	1	1	2	1	1	1
10	Broward	4	3	1	--	3	1	1	*
11	Dade	1 H	5 H	-	1	--		1	1
12	Volusia	4	NA	*	--	3	1	1	1 CHS
13	Citrus	3	4	*	1	1	--	1	1
14	Polk	2	***	2	NA	3	1	*	--
15	Martin	7	--	3	--	4	1	1	1

Notes: * Could not be completed due to lack of consents or participation.
*** We met with the group and input was obtained via survey.
– Was not completed for various reasons (e.g., time constraints, change in personnel).
AA = African American participants.
H = Hispanic participants.
CHS = Children's Home Society.
NA = No active group or organization in county.

total cases of 1 percent experienced between 1995 and 1997. This is a rapid and significant increase in the number of children requiring state care.

Licensed Capacity

The total number of children that may be cared for in licensed homes (licensed capacity) increased from 13,000 in 1989 to a high of more than 17,000 at the end of 1999. A large increase in the licensed capacity occurred between 1989 and 1994-95, followed by a more gradual increase in 1998-99.

In summary, there has been a gradual and steady increase in the licensing capacity in the State, but for the first time in five years the capacity in 1998-99 lagged behind the number of foster children needing care.

FIGURE 1. Total Foster Care Caseload in Florida, 1995-1999

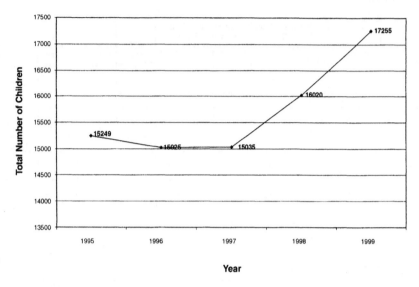

Total Number of Licenses

The number of licenses issued to foster homes in Florida over the past 10 years rose from 4100 at the beginning of 1989 to approximately 5600 at the end of 1999. As Figure 2 reveals, there was a dramatic increase from the 1989-90 period through the 1994-95 period. This increase slowed during the next five years, and there was less change during the 1998-99 period than at any time since 1989.

In summary, there has been a trend toward an increased number of licenses that has now stabilized or is slightly decreasing. According to Department staff, this trend has led to increases in the number of children that current foster homes are licensed to serve, and increased over-crowding. Evidence of this trend was provided in the meetings we held with foster parents and agency staff. Many agencies are routinely requesting waivers to exceed the 5-child limit rule because no additional homes are available.

Length of Stay

Figure 3 shows that the average length of stay in foster care remained relatively stable over the past five years. The mean number of months in

FIGURE 2. Number of Licensed Homes in Florida, 1989-1999

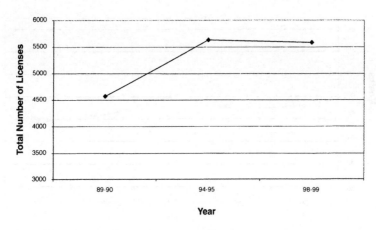

care in 1995 was approximately 37, and there were very small increases or decreases over the years, ending with a mean stay of approximately 36 months in 1999. When the length of stay is broken down by other factors, such as age and racial category, some important differences emerge.

Length of Stay by Age. Figure 4 shows the length of stay in foster care by age group. The oldest group of those in care (19 and older) had the longest stays of any group at each of the five years described. The mean length of stay for this group in 1995 and 1996 was relatively steady (ranging from 78 to 82 months), increasing to approximately 87 months in 1997 and 92 months in 1998. These increases were followed by a decline in 1999 to a mean of approximately 83 months in care.

The next three age groups (16-18, 13-15, and 6-12) showed patterns over time that were similar to each other. The length of stay was rather steady over the entire period, with small increases and decreases. The three trend lines fan out slightly over the five-year span, indicating that the differences between the age groups are growing very slightly.

The youngest group, aged 0-5, had the shortest average length of stay over the five-year period of all age groups. The mean stay in care was approximately 22 months in 1995, which slowly and steadily declined to a low point of 18 months in 1999.

In summary, most age groups showed little change over the five-year period. The oldest group of children in care stayed the longest, and in spite of a large decrease from 1998 to 1999, still had a slightly longer average length of stay than in 1995. The youngest group of children in care had the shortest length of stay, and the average has actually de-

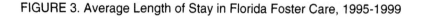

FIGURE 3. Average Length of Stay in Florida Foster Care, 1995-1999

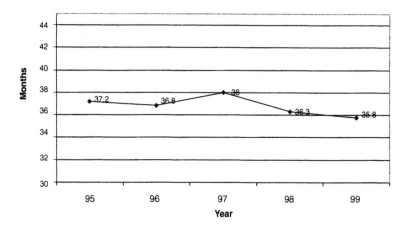

creased in the past year. Those in the middle age groups have remained stable over the past five years.

Length of Stay by Race. Length of stay in foster care varied during the past five years depending upon racial category (African American, White, and Other) (see Figure 5). The data collected by the Department of Children and Families did not permit any other partitioning by race or ethnicity. African American children had consistently longer average lengths of stay at each of the five previous years. There was an increase in 1997, but the length of stay has remained fairly constant, at approximately 40-42 months. White children also showed a steady average length of stay, but much shorter (approximately 32 months in 1995), and there was a gradual decline to approximately 29 months by 1999. Those children included in the "Other" racial category had a similar average length of stay to the White children in 1995, but there was a decline over the five years to a low of 20 months in 1999. In summary, in 1999 the average stay for those in the "Other" category was 20 months shorter than for African American children and 10 months shorter than for White children. These trends have particular relevance to the findings of the study related to children feeling powerless and remaining in care too long.

Foster Children Views

A consistent theme noted by children in foster care was that they thought some parents were dedicated to giving children in need a good

FIGURE 4. Average Length of Stay in Foster Care in Florida by Age Group, 1995-1999

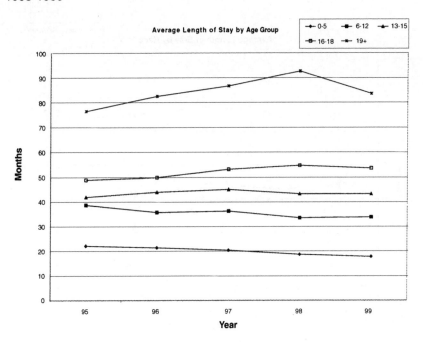

home and support. They remarked that parents wanted to provide positive experiences to children. Foster children also reported that monetary concerns played a major role in people choosing to foster or staying in foster parenting. They thought some parents went into foster care because they needed the money or, once they had become foster parents, they became dependent upon the money and could not stop fostering. It was noted by some teens that they were aware of the amount of money allotted to their family and felt that their needs were not covered appropriately given the amount received by the family. The majority of the children interviewed reinforced the views of the foster parents. Both groups were consistent about the need for more money for school activities, special needs, clothing allowance, and other incidentals experienced by most children.

The foster children interviewed focused many of their concerns on the lack of attention and support that they received from Department staff and the lack of trust they felt with the staff. They felt this had a major effect on the retention of foster parents. Generally they felt sup-

FIGURE 5. Average Length of Stay in Foster Care in Florida by Race, 1995-1999

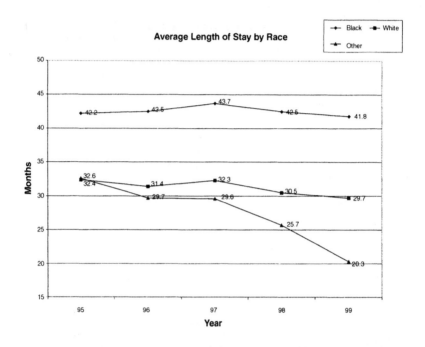

ported by their foster parents, but they felt that counselors often did not do their jobs. They described failure on the part of counselors to provide support, citing infrequent visits by the counselors, and not providing promised transportation. Support to foster children and their foster parents was very important to the families. Many of the foster teenagers felt that it was critical to have access to their counselors on a 24-hour basis so that problems could be addressed rapidly. They felt fearful when they had no one to call in the event of a problematic home situation.

Foster children reiterated the concern of foster parents (addressed in the study report submitted to the Department of Children and Families) (Jarmon, Mathiesen, Clarke, McCulloch, & Lazear, 2000) that foster children need more effective ways to communicate with their foster care counselor. They also indicated that their freedom to communicate is sometimes restricted by foster parents, in spite of regulations that assure the ability to maintain contact. For example, a foster parent may attempt to control a teenage foster child by restricting phone privileges, which also serves to limit access to the counselor.

Another issue many foster children and foster parents raised was the length of time in placement. Many children had been in foster care for three or more years with no permanency plan in place. They did not understand how the rules on placing children could be so blatantly broken and why the courts took so long to make a decision about their lives. The general concern was that the system moves too slowly in securing foster children's stability and a plan for the future.

Many of the foster children also reported wanting a greater role in the selection of their foster home. They thought that they should be given more information when they are being taken from their parents to reduce the guilt and fear that they felt when being pulled from the home, and they wanted to have a voice in the type of foster home chosen. Consistently, foster children and parents talked about the emotional upheaval foster children experienced when they were taken from their homes, placed in a home without information, and then moved without much explanation or rationale. Foster children and parents felt that whenever a child is moved, they should have regular contact with a caseworker or counselor to help them through this transition, and if they are old enough, they should be given more information about why they are being moved and the location to where they are being moved.

The foster children in the study were also quite frank about the ways that other foster children used the system. They knew how difficult some foster children could be and they knew that foster parents were unable to punish them in meaningful ways. This frustrated some because they wanted to see limits put on some foster children who disturbed the families. They also were sympathetic with their foster parents and did not want to see good foster parents manipulated by foster children or the system.

The teenagers in the study clearly understood how "fatigued" and burned out foster parents could become. Some suggested that the Department should give foster parents more praise. *"They are braver than most people."*

Foster teens felt strongly about having a voice in the foster care system, including having a voice in recruiting new foster families. They wanted to do outreach and meet the families that are interested in fostering. These teens thought that they could help screen out the parents who may not be good foster parents. They also felt that there should be a better way to screen for prospective foster parents. One foster child recommended that the Department invite selected families to become foster parents. One type of family they would target is one in which a parent was formerly a foster child.

The foster children also felt strongly that in order to have enough foster families, the Department needed to appreciate current foster parents by regularly recognizing them and giving them respect. There were many ideas offered such as having annual dinners, prizes, additional funds, providing babysitting and similar supports to foster parents who are rarely given any appreciation or gifts of thanks. This recognition of current foster parents would help recruitment because, as the teens put it, *"Word of mouth is effective in recruitment."* If the parents are supported then they will share their positive experiences with other foster parents. The foster children also recommended the use of newspapers and radio announcements.

Recommendations made by some of the youths interviewed were:

- Foster children should have the opportunity to meet foster parents before they are placed.
- There should be access to a phone at all times so those children feel safe and able to report problems.
- Siblings should be placed in one home if at all possible, and should always have the opportunity to visit regularly if not placed together.
- There should be special efforts made to minimize identification of foster children at school (e.g., workers coming to the school and pulling them out of class).
- The money ($50) that is allotted for clothing for a first time placement does not address the needs of children who are moved. The clothing is often left at the original placement, leaving the child without needed items.
- Foster children prefer foster family homes to group homes.
- The foster adolescents themselves would like to be involved in the recruitment process.

DISCUSSION

Implications for Family Social Work Practice

This report and the following conclusions reflect a careful analysis of a vast amount of information provided to study researchers from focus groups, interviews, and survey responses on the broad issues of recruitment and retention. Virtually all strategies proposed in this report were based on comments and suggestions from the voices of the children themselves. Not surprisingly, many of the ideas were the same as those suggested in national studies of foster care. A broader, more detailed report is available from the Department of Children and Families, entitled Florida Foster Care Recruitment and Retention Project (Jarmon et al., 2000); however, the focus on the "voices" of the children has implications for family social work practitioners, policy makers, and those interested in enhancing services to foster children.

1. *Foster children feel powerless, unsupported and do not trust the foster care system. Many children are in foster care many years longer than they should be and some experience many foster home moves, making it difficult for them to feel secure.* Family social workers must consider the impact of years in the child welfare system as they address the issues presented by both foster parents and the foster children themselves, and make efforts to be in contact with DCF counselors to coordinate efforts on behalf of the child.

2. *The foster care administrative system should be redesigned to assure that foster children are given adequate and on-going support by their counselors when they are placed. Also, it is important to identify ways the children can contact Department staff when they have urgent needs, such as emotional or physical needs, or to maintain a healthy lifestyle. There should be limits on the number of counselors that foster families are required to contact.* For family social workers, this implies ongoing interaction with DCF counselors to minimize misunderstandings and overlap, and to maximize the chance of children receiving prompt and comprehensive treatment.

3. *The foster care system and courts must become more efficient in meeting the needs of foster children, with emphasis on achieving permanency as quickly as possible.* While there is legislative support for the development of permanency plans, many children have experienced delays. Those working with foster families and their foster children must remain aware of timelines so that there is sufficient time to aid in the transition to the permanency plan. Family social workers can also serve in an advocacy role for the prompt resolution of the plan.

4. *Give foster children more information and counseling about what is happening to them when they are moved.* Family social workers can play an important part of a team approach with DCF counsel-

ors when a child is also being seen in therapy, as they can remain as trusted persons who are not determining placement status.

5. *Provide 24-hour hot line numbers to foster children for their use only in the emergencies involving their treatment at their foster home.* This can also be an area of advocacy for family social workers. The importance of empowerment of the foster child, and the importance of a good match for family and child can be used as proximal goals in treatment.

6. *Give older foster children a choice of foster homes prior to placement.* As teens move to independent living, this may be an appropriate part of the process, and family social workers are in the position to facilitate the transition.

7. *Insure that foster parents are culturally sensitive and culturally competent before placing a child from a different culture with them.* All members of the team need to be trained and competent regarding diversity issues of all kinds, and work toward identifying potential foster parents. Family social workers are needed to provide input to agencies regarding the appropriateness of placement from their perspective. Often a child has had multiple placements with foster families, and the goal of all members of the team, after safety is assured, is to be sensitive to the unique needs of each child in each transition.

Effective practitioners recognize the need to listen carefully to the voices of those at the center of the enormous child welfare system, and move beyond important safety issues, which must be paramount. From a systems perspective, each part can influence and is influenced by the other parts. All members of the team must be aware of the events that impact the foster family and their charges. Developing a cohesive and responsive system that works efficiently in the best interests of the child will keep current foster parents engaged and rewarded, and will attract new foster parents that will assure that the search for family is a successful one for each child in need.

REFERENCES

Administration for Children, Youth and Families (2000). Protecting the well being of children (Update June, 2000). Available: <http://www.acf.dhhs.gov/programs>.
American Academy of Pediatrics, Committee on Early Childhood, Adoption and Dependent Care (1994). Health care of children in foster care. *Pediatrics, 93* (2), 1-4.

Babb, A.L. (1999). *Ethics in American adoption.* Westport, Connecticut: Bergin & Garvey.

Berrick, J.D., Courtney, M.E., & Barth, R.P. (1993). Specialized foster care and group home care: Similarities and differences in the characteristics of children in care. *Children and Youth Services Review, 15,* 453-475.

Child Welfare League of America (2000). National factsheet. Available: <http://www. cwla.org/publicpolicy>.

Epstein, W.M. (1999). *Children who could have been: The legacy of child welfare in wealthy America.* Madison, Wisconsin: University of Wisconsin Press.

Fanshel, D., Finch, S., & Grundy, J. (1989). Modes of exit from foster family care and adjustment at time of departure of children with unstable life histories. *Child Welfare, 68* (4), 391-401.

Hernandez, D.J. (1993). *America's children: Resources from family, government, and the economy.* New York: Russell Sage.

Jarmon, B.J., Mathiesen, S.G., Clarke, L., McCulloch, E., & Lazear, K. (2000) *Foster Care Recruitment and Retention Perspectives of Stakeholders on the Critical Factors Affecting Recruitment and Retention of Foster Parents.* Unpublished report submitted to the State of Florida Department of Children and Families and the Lawton and Rhea Chiles Center for Healthy Mothers and Babies. Tallahassee, FL.

Klee, L., & Halfon, N. (1987). Mental health care for foster children in California. *Child Abuse and Neglect, 15* (1), 63-74.

McIntyre, A., & Keesler, T.Y. (1986). Psychological disorders among foster children. *Journal of Clinical Child Psychology, 15* (4), 297-303.

Schor, E.L. (1982). The foster care system and health status of foster children. *Pediatrics, 69* (5), 521-528.

State of Florida Department of Health and Rehabilitative Services, (1989). *Performance audit of the foster care program.* Tallahassee, FL: Florida Department of Health and Rehabilitative Services.

United States Department of Health and Human Services, Children's Bureau (1999). *Guidelines for public policy and state legislation governing permanence for children.* Washington, DC: Author.

United States General Accounting Office (1989). *Children and youths: About 68,000 homeless and 186,000 in shared housing at any given time.* Washington, D.C.: Author.

United States General Accounting Office (1989). *Foster parents: Recruiting and pre-service training practices needs evaluation.* GAO/HRD-89-86. Washington, D.C.: Author.

Zuravin, S.J., Benedict, M., & Somerfield M. (1997). Child maltreatment in family foster care: Foster home correlates. In J.D. Berrick, R. Barth, and N. Gilbert (Eds.), *Child Welfare Research Review, Vol. 2.* New York: Columbia University Press.

Family Involvement and Schizophrenia: A Developmental Model

Sally G. Mathiesen, PhD

SUMMARY. This paper presents the Family Involvement and Schizo-phrenia model, an adaptation of Rolland's Family Systems/Illness model (1994). Rolland's model conceptualized the development of the individ-ual, family, and illness in psychosocial terms using adult developmental theory and family life cycle concepts. The Family Involvement and Schizophrenia Model builds on this prior work, and consists of (1) a psychosocial typology of illness based on characteristics often associ-ated with a diagnosis of schizophrenia, and which are hypothesized to impact individual development and family relationships and (2) the changing psychosocial demands and family relationships at different phases of the illness, which represent an integration of the age-linked stages of individual development with the fluctuations in family cohesion over the life cycle. The Family Involvement and Schizophrenia model will enable clinicians, researchers, and families to conceptualize changing family relationships, and to target individuals and families at greatest stress points in order to provide more individualized treatment over the life cycle. *[Article copies available for a fee from The Haworth Document Delivery Service: 1-800-342-9678. E-mail address: <getinfo@haworthpressinc.com> Website: <http://www.HaworthPress.com> © 2001 by The Haworth Press, Inc. All rights reserved.]*

Sally G. Mathiesen is affiliated with Florida State University, School of Social Work.

This research was supported by the National Institute of Mental Health, (NIMH) Grant # RO3-MH 56298-01.

[Haworth co-indexing entry note]: "Family Involvement and Schizophrenia: A Developmental Model." Mathiesen, Sally G. Co-published simultaneously in *Journal of Family Social Work* (The Haworth Social Work Practice Press, an imprint of The Haworth Press, Inc.) Vol. 6, No. 1, 2001, pp. 35-52; and: *Families and Health: Cross-Cultural Perspectives* (ed: Jorge Delva) The Haworth Social Work Practice Press, an imprint of The Haworth Press, Inc., 2001, pp. 35-52. Single or multiple copies of this article are available for a fee from The Haworth Document Delivery Service [1-800-342-9678, 9:00 a.m. - 5:00 p.m. (EST). E-mail address: getinfo@haworthpressinc.com].

KEYWORDS. Schizophrenia, family involvement, psychosocial typology, developmental model

INTRODUCTION

The increasingly important role of the family in the treatment of schizophrenia has a long and varied history. The family has been seen as a causal factor in the illness (Fromm-Reichman, 1950; Lidz & Lidz, 1949), a source of stress capable of affecting the course of the illness (Brown, Birley, & Wing, 1972; Vaughn & Leff, 1976), a resource and advocate for policy change (Bernheim, 1990), and in need of support due to the burdens of caregiving (National Institute of Mental Health [NIMH], 1991; Lefley, 1989; Falloon, Boyd, & McGill, 1984; Group for the Advancement of Psychiatry [GAP], 1992; Bulger, Wandersman, & Goldman, 1993). In 1992 the Clinical Research Services Panel of NIMH recommended that the various kinds and degree of family involvement should be "an important variable in rehabilitation effectiveness research" (Attkisson, Cook, Karno, Lehman, McGlashan, Meltzer, O'Connor, Richardson, Rosenblatt, Wells, & Williams, 1992, p. 601).

In a review of the literature, Yank and colleagues (1993) described vulnerability-stress models of schizophrenia as incorporating a variety of etiological components (biological, developmental, learning, genetic, and environmental) which interact to produce a degree of vulnerability (Zubin & Spring, 1977; Goldstein, 1990; Nuechterlein, 1987; Nuechterlein & Dawson, 1984). The vulnerability represents the risk of relapse or acute episode. Environmental stress impacts a vulnerable person, resulting in a schizophrenic episode (Straube & Oades, 1992).

A systems perspective is evident in these conceptualizations, which have considered the mediating factors in schizophrenia (Anthony & Liberman, 1986; Ciompi, 1988; 1989; Nicholson & Neufeld, 1992; Strauss, 1989). The models emphasize "interactions over time, feedback processes, biological functioning, stressful events, cognitive processes, coping skills, competence, and symptomatology" (Yank et al., 1993, p. 56).

Most psychosocial treatments for the severely mentally ill are based on the vulnerability-stress theory, with the goal of reducing stress for the vulnerable individual. Psychosocial treatments that intervene at the environmental level to reduce stress, such as family interventions, have been shown to have a positive effect on the subsequent course of schizophrenic illness (Anderson et al., 1980; 1986; Leff et al., 1982; 1985;

Goldstein et al., 1978; Goldstein, 1984; Falloon et al., 1984; Hogarty et al., 1986; 1991; Barrowclough & Tarrier, 1990; McFarlane et al., 1993). In addition, researchers have articulated the need for longitudinal studies to determine the changing patterns of the illness (Ciompi, 1987; Wynne, 1988; Carpenter et al., 1990; GAP, 1992; Belitsky & McGlashan, 1993). It is critical to systematically investigate patterns of family involvement across the life cycle and to ultimately use the information to target treatment more effectively.

But there are several critical issues in regard to our knowledge about schizophrenia and the interaction with family that have important clinical and research implications: (1) Family interventions have been conducted almost exclusively with individuals who were hospitalized or resided with their family. There is little longitudinal information to characterize patterns of family involvement for those living in the community; (2) There are no existing comprehensive models to predict how family interaction patterns may change over the course of the illness; (3) Client characteristics, such as gender, ethnicity, and age, have been shown to be related to the course of illness, but little is understood of their relation to family involvement.

The purpose of this paper is to present the Family Involvement and Schizophrenia (FIS) model, a developmental model of the individual, family, and course of schizophrenia in psychosocial terms. Rolland's Family Systems/Illness Model (1994), developed primarily for chronic physical illness and disability, was adapted to address the demands commonly associated with a diagnosis of schizophrenia. The FIS model provides a comprehensive, longitudinal, developmental view of the illness. It will enable clinicians, researchers, and families to conceptualize changing family relationships, and to target individuals and families at greatest stress points in order to provide more individualized treatment over the life cycle.

FAMILY INVOLVEMENT
AND SCHIZOPHRENIA (FIS) MODEL

Building on the work of Rolland (1994), the FIS model consists of (1) a psychosocial typology, based on characteristics often associated with a diagnosis of schizophrenia, and which are hypothesized to impact individual development and family relationships; (2) the changing psychosocial demands and family relationships at different phases of the illness, which represent an integration of the age-linked stages of individual development (Levinson, 1978; 1986) with the fluctuations in family cohesion over the life cycle (Combrinck-Graham (1985). The resulting FIS model is an integrated conceptual model that depicts the undulating course of normative family interaction patterns, and the hypothesized effect of a diagnosed schizophrenic illness.

The psychosocial typology of schizophrenia from the Family Involvement and Schizophrenia (FIS) model will be presented first, followed by the phases of illness and the transitions between them. Next, the theoretical relationship between the age-linked stages of individual development, combined with the fluctuations in family cohesion over the phases of illness is presented.

Psychosocial Typology of Schizophrenia

The typology of the FIS model is based on the psychosocial demands that are imposed on the individual and family by variations in onset, course, gender, variation in outcome, level of incapacitation, and phase of illness. The categories are hypothesized to be those most relevant to the psychosocial issues posed by chronic conditions, and also related to the developmental tasks at different phases of the illness.

Onset

The FIS model includes both the timing (early to late) and the trajectory (acute to insidious) of onset. Rolland (1994) included only acute or gradual onset in his theoretical model, and distinctions were made in relation to the presentation of symptomatology, not necessarily biological development. He posited that illnesses with gradual onset require readjustment of the family structure, roles, and coping styles over a protracted period, while acute onset require the same adaptations in a compressed time period. Similarly, the rate or trajectory of onset (acute or insidious) has been included in the FIS model, as it represents an essential parameter in identifying course types in schizophrenia (Marengo, 1994), and has been used in long-term follow-up studies (Bleuler, 1978; Ciompi, 1980; Krauz et al., 1993).

The FIS model incorporates the additional category of the timing of onset (early or late) as an important modification. "Age of onset is the single most important clue to the etiology of (schizophrenic) illness" (DeLisi, 1992, p. 212), and two distinct times of onset have been identified. The differences in the developmental disruptions between early onset, where brain defects affecting language processing are likely, and late onset, where recovery from acute episodes may be easier due to fewer developmental deficits, are important aspects of the illness that need further research (DeLisi, 1992). The DSM-IIIR (American Psychiatric Association, 1987) allowed a diagnosis of schizophrenia to be made after age 45, defined as late-onset patients (DeLisi, 1992). Clinical research found fewer negative symptoms in persons with late onset schizophrenia than in early onset (Yassa & Suranyll-Cadotte, 1993). Including the age of onset into the typology will facilitate a systematic approach for research designs and interpretation of findings, as well as assist the clinician in targeting intervention approaches.

Course of Illness

The FIS model consists of three aspects of the course of illness: the type of course (progressive, constant, or relapsing/episodic), the level of incapacitation in role functioning (including functioning in the areas of social relationships, work, and self-care), and patterns of psychotic and residual symptoms.

The courses of illness as described by Rolland (1994) were consistent with the course variation in schizophrenia. Progressive illnesses are those that are continually symptomatic and increasing in severity. Constant courses are those in which there is an initial event, followed by a stabilized condition. The residual effect is a semipermanent deficit predictable over long time periods. Relapsing courses are characterized by relatively symptom-free periods of varying length alternating with periods of exacerbation. The continual uncertainty as to when the next family crisis will occur, combined with the strains of the crises themselves, make this course of illness uniquely stressful and psychologically challenging, regardless of the degree of biological severity.

In the FIS, the role-functioning dimension was added to the typology. The patterns of role functioning in the domains of social interaction, work, and self-care are included in the diagnosis of schizophrenia, as well as representing important areas for determining treatment efficacy (Heinrichs et al., 1984; Marengo, 1994). Their independence from symptomatology levels is indicative of the heterogeneity and complexity of patterns in the course of the illness. The inclusion of a role-functioning dimension contributes valuable information to the long-term course of the illness.

Patterns of psychotic and residual symptoms each represent unique stressors and necessary adaptations that affect the objective and subjective experience of the illness. Rolland discussed variables that were implicated in the adaptation to illness, but were not included in a separate category, such as the visibility of symptoms (visible symptoms increase social stigma, but allow for more objective interactions with the patient than invisible symptoms, which increase ambiguity for the family). Visibility of symptoms is an area that is so central to the individual and family that it should be included in any typology attempting to chart the course of the illness (Marengo, 1994). By utilizing the constant, progressive, and relapsing categories, in combination with the role-functioning and symptom subcategories, course types can be more systematically and sensitively investigated.

Gender

The FIS model added gender to the psychosocial typology outlined by Rolland (1994). This is an important contribution, as there is research that suggests that gender has implications for the developmental perspective in schizophrenia. One study found that young men appeared to be more at risk for a poor outcome than young women (Leventhal et al., 1984). The authors contend that men tend to have more difficulty in the early developmental stages due to limitations related to schooling, socialization, or independent living. In a summary of gender-specific data, Bardenstein and McGlashan (1990) noted that women, in general, required lower doses of medication, had fewer relapses, and were less prone to suicide and comorbidity of psychiatric illnesses than men with schizophrenia.

There is evidence that women may not display the same type of illness plateau as men (Group for the Advancement of Psychiatry [GAP], 1992). Women may require more adjustment in the later stage, such as during parenthood or menopause. Better outcomes for women in the past may have been related to their increased tendency to be married and to have a spouse and/or children to assist them in their illness. Other evidence suggests that young women with schizophrenia are not as likely to be married, but they may still be a parent. Loss of parental rights due to illness, or remaining childless may increase the stress in later developmental stages of schizophrenia (Salonkongas, 1983; Seeman, 1986). Viewing the limited gender-specific data in a developmental perspective highlights the need for a comprehensive model that incorporates critical psychosocial variables over the life cycle so that relationships may be tested.

Variation in Outcome

In the FIS model, a useful description of the heterogeneity in schizophrenia is the variation in outcome over time, ranging from deterioration to improvement. While Rolland's model included the categories of Fatal, Possibly fatal/Shortened lifespan, and Nonfatal, it is important to make distinctions between physical illness and outcomes associated with a diagnosis of schizophrenia. Schizophrenia is not in itself a fatal illness, but it does result in "an increased risk of suicide, physical illness, and early death" in comparison to the general population (GAP, 1992, p. 5). Estimates of 5 percent to 10 percent suicide rates, and a lifespan shortened by up to 10 years have been reported (GAP, 1992). The results are in part due to the lack of optimal care for the population, and the growing numbers of homeless chronically mentally ill in major urban centers (Talbott, 1990).

For the family, their initial expectation of the degree of loss may have the most impact, and yet these perceptions may be based on inaccurate information (Rolland, 1994). The primary difference among outcome types was the degree to which the family anticipated loss and its effect on the family. Illnesses that are known to be fatal result in less ambiguity than those that may shorten life. Using existing long-term studies of schizophrenia as a basis for hypotheses, and the onset and course categories in the typology as variables, a psychosocial picture of the course of illness will begin to emerge that may be used to provide more accurate prognostic information to the individual and family.

The FIS model considers the degree of uncertainty/predictability in the nature of the illness or the rate of change as a metacharacteristic that influences all the other factors. The greater the degree of uncertainty of outcome, the greater the need for flexible problem-solving styles and contingency plans (Rolland, 1994). The overarching quality of the degree of uncertainty or predictability in schizophrenia is particularly a function of the state of knowledge that is possessed currently. There are many aspects of the long-term course of schizophrenia that are undiscovered, increasing the level of stress and anxiety for all those affected by the illness. Knowledge of both the rate of change and the nature of the illness are incomplete. But recognition of the limitations in these areas enables a clinician to alert the individual and family to possible changes in the illness, and the changing psychosocial demands and expectations as the illness moves from one phase to another. As described in the introduction to the model, the following section will address the second part of the FIS model: the phases of illness, and the transitions between the phases.

Phases of Illness

Each phase of illness demands "significantly different strengths, attitudes, or changes from a family" (Rolland, 1994, p. 43). The phases are very compatible with researchers' descriptions of the eras or "epochs" of schizophrenia over time (Carpenter & Kirkpatrick, 1988). The FIS model modified the phases for the demands of schizophrenia, and are described below.

Early Phase

The crisis (early) phase includes both the beginning of psychotic symptoms and early treatment, and the prodromal period that precedes symptomatology. The main tasks for the individual and family are to engage in short term crisis reorganization, grieve for the loss of prior family image, and understand the developmental aspects of the illness.

Mid Phase

The mid phase (chronic course) includes periods of active psychosis and nonpsychotic periods between episodes. Family and individual psychosocial tasks include developing a normal family life in face of the uncertainty and limits of illness, and preserve maximum autonomy for all members.

Late Phase

The terminal phase is re-labeled the "late phase" in the FIS model. The late phase (third epoch) refers to late course and outcome, when some patients improve and others stabilize or deteriorate (Carpenter & Kirkpatrick, 1988). Contrary to earlier conceptions, many patients with schizophrenia show sustained and substantial improvement in psychopathology late in the course of illness (Lin & Kleinman, 1988; GAP, 1992). Acceptance of changing generational roles, physiological changes and losses, and learning to define a new balance between youth and age are the primary developmental tasks.

The changing needs of the family over the life span must be considered in a developmental context, as family interaction patterns may differentially affect the individual with schizophrenia at different stages. Due in part to the failure to achieve or maintain adult roles, the impact on self-esteem, and the disruption in family relationships, many young adults diagnosed with schizophrenia engage in self-destructive behaviors, contributing to the perception that treatment is resisted or refused (Pepper & Ryglewicz, 1984). The focus on the early years, when safety and support are critical, may have contributed to the dearth of information about other stages of life. Little is known about the life of the individual and family affected by schizophrenia in mid-life, and some writers have posited that it may be the most opportune period for intervention, rather than a time for less intensive efforts (GAP, 1992). The mid-adulthood years may represent a time for re-examination of strengths and limitations, and an openness to change.

The results of a review of long term follow-up studies indicate that the virulent effects of the illness subside to a great degree in middle-age, and reach a plateau or even gradual improvement with time (McGlashan & Carpenter, 1988). Research attention should be focused on the middle and late phases, as little is known about the years beyond early adulthood, which comprise the majority of a person's life with schizophrenia. Progressive, or episodic in nature, as the individual and family adapt to the realities of daily life with chronic illness.

Transition Periods

The time periods between the three phases described are important in themselves, and represent critical points of leverage in adaptation. When issues remain unresolved from previous phases, the next transition can become very difficult.

According to Rolland's conceptualization, the move from crisis to chronic is the most difficult transition to negotiate and the most significant in terms of the ability of the family to reevaluate their coping and adaptation. A family that became competent at marshalling resources and drawing together as a family in a crisis phase may find the same behaviors maladaptive in the chronic phase (Rolland, 1994). The transition from mid to late phase involves evolving from day-to-day coping to expression of affect, and reevaluation of changing roles.

Integration of Individual Development and Family Spiral Theories

Rolland's model drew on the adult developmental perspective as explicated by Levinson (1978; 1986), as well as the fluctuating levels of family cohesion described by Combrinck-Graham (1985) to combine the three paths of individual, family, and illness development. As adapted to schizophrenia, these theoretical constructs must be integrated to provide a baseline for further theory development and testing.

Figure 1 represents the Family Involvement and Schizophrenia model. The following sections will further describe the theoretical foundations for the model.

Age-Linked Stages of Adult Development

Rolland (1994) applied Levinson's (1978; 1986) individual adult theory of life structure to the family. Levinson's model provides distinct, age-linked developmental eras for the entire life cycle, and emphasizes the importance of transitions from one era to the next. His hypothesis for the underlying order of the human life cycle was based on empirical studies he conducted with men and women, and was meant to provide a starting point for individual variation in life course as a result of the influences of biology, personality, culture, social roles, and life events. The following section closely follows Levinson's description of the four eras of his theory (Levinson, 1986).

Levinson delineated four periods in life structure development, each lasting approximately twenty years, and each era is preceded by a critical transition stage. The goal of the transition period is to carefully

FIGURE 1

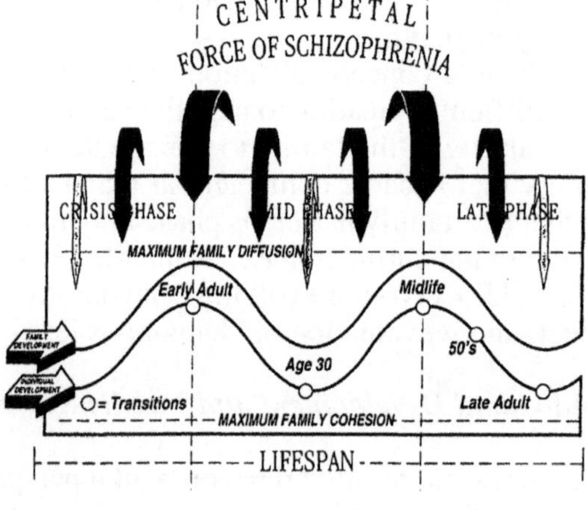

weigh different options for the individual and the family, which will serve as a plan for the next life cycle phase. Transitions from one phase to the next are the points at which individuals and families are the most vulnerable, due to the task of reevaluation of previous life structures.

Preadulthood Era (birth through age 22). The primary task in childhood and adolescence is to establish the distinction between "me" and "not me" as the individual separates from family and other aspects of the preadult world. Although this era represents great and rapid biopsychosocial growth, in the context of the life cycle it is a basis from which to begin further development.

Early Adulthood Era (age 17-45). This era is preceded by the Early Adult Transition (17-22), which requires that the newly merging adult modify family, peer, and other social relationships, and begin to create a niche in the adult world. Early adulthood can be the time of greatest reward and also of greatest stress. The individual must pursue early goals, define a distinct place in society, raise a family, and assume a more "senior" position as an adult. A transition period around age 30 is a time for reappraisal of the life structure, and preparation for the final segment of early adulthood.

Middle Adulthood Era (ages 40-65). The Midlife Transition (40-45) results in an appreciable change in lifestyle as early adulthood is left behind. Successful resolution of conflicts regarding the growing awareness of one's mortality and limitations can lead to increased compassion, empathy, and inner peace, while an unsuccessful transition may result in an increasingly stagnant and unproductive life (Levinson, 1986). In the middle adulthood era, taking responsibility for one's own work and maintaining "senior member" status of that self-created world is the paramount task. A transition around age 50 allows for mid-era modification of middle adulthood.

Late Adulthood Era (ages 60-80+). The Late Adult Transition (60-65) precedes the Late Adulthood Era, and is the result of the gradual recognition and experience of physical decline and the culturally-defined change of generation in the 60s to "old age." The developmental task of this era is to end an earlier life structure and find an appropriate balance between the energy, interests and inner resources of youth and age. The loss of "center stage" must give way to a new involvement with society and the self.

Family Spiral Model

The Family Spiral Model (Combrinck-Graham, 1985) depicts three generations of a family alternating through the life cycle between eras of high cohesion (centripetal) and lower family cohesion (centrifugal). Ideally, the periods coincide with family developmental tasks that require similar levels of cohesion (Rolland, 1994). The concept of centrifugal (pushing away from center) and centripetal (moving toward the center) forces operating at different points in the family life cycle is useful in combining the individual, family, and illness developmental process (Beavers & Voeller, 1983; Combrinck-Graham, 1985).

The concept describes the "goodness of fit" between developmental tasks and the relative need for internal and group cohesive energy to accomplish the tasks. For example, during the family life cycle period of child rearing, the individual and the family have a life structure that emphasizes the solidarity of family life. The "pull" is inward, and centripetal forces allow outside boundaries to be strengthened, while boundaries between family members become more diffuse, as the family operates as a unit. As the family transitions to a centrifugal period such as adolescence, individual and family developmental tasks require a loosening of the external boundaries. An outward "push" away from center occurs, and individual boundaries between family members become more defined in response to developmental tasks (Rolland, 1994).

Rolland theorized that illness and disability exert an inward pull or centripetal force upon individual and family members, and will vary according to the illness type and phase. The onset of a chronic illness is seen as the addition of a new member of the family, setting the stage for a period of high cohesion. "Symptoms, loss of function, the demands of shifting or new illness-related roles, and the fear of loss through death all serve to make a family turn inward" (Rolland, 1994, p. 109). If the onset of a chronic illness occurs at a centrifugal point in the family life, the family may be derailed. The individual and family members' autonomy is placed at great risk due to the new demands for cohesion due to illness coinciding with naturally lower demands of a centrifugal phase. If the onset of a chronic illness occurs at a point in the life cycle which requires greater cohesion (centripetal), there is a risk that the pull of the illness and the pull of the life cycle phase will amplify each other (Rolland, 1994). At best, the centripetal period will be prolonged; at worst, the family may become frozen at this stage and become enmeshed. Other families may survive the initial stage, but when faced with the developmental changes of adolescence, for example, the long-standing and rigid patterns of cohesion clash with the need for autonomy, and the family system may break down.

FIS MODEL AS A FRAMEWORK FOR ASSESSMENT
AND INTERVENTION

The combination of the typology of schizophrenia in psychosocial terms, combined with the phases of the illness and the developmental processes of the individual and family provides a basis for assessment and guide to intervention. The model emphasizes the changing "goodness of fit" between individual, family, and illness development over the course of the illness.

For example, a course of illness categorized by the FIS typology as relapsing would require multiple adjustments for the individual and the family. Relapsing illnesses alternate between requirements for greater family cohesion, and periods of release from the demands of the illness (Rolland, 1994). The degree of uncertainty as to when the individual and family may need to shift to another mode tends to keep some members of the family in a centripetal mode, even when the ill member is asymptomatic.

The time of onset is critical to a developmental concept, as the illness will force a family into a transition period that is characterized by the family task of adapting to possible loss or deterioration. If the onset occurs when a family is already in a transitional period, the intensity of previously unresolved issues will be magnified. There is an increased risk of the illness being inappropriately ignored or becoming the sole focus of the next developmental stage.

The phases of the illness will have an impact on the fluctuating levels of cohesion with family. The early phase, requiring high cohesion, is analogous to the childhood era. The mid phase, whose primary task is to establish autonomy within the restrictions of the illness, is much like adolescence and adulthood, with less cohesion required. The late phase corresponds to that of later life, during which a return to family occurs as a result of physical decline and increased caregiving tasks (Rolland, 1994).

The categories of the typology and the changing demands of the illness can help to focus the clinician's approach with the family in the early phase, clarifying treatment planning and goal-setting. The structure also is valuable to the individual and family who may be unfamiliar with the mental health system, and may be overwhelmed by the potential impact on all their lives. Describing the normative developmental landmarks and tasks of the individual and family, combined with the additional psychosocial tasks that may be required over time allows for preparation for future transitions. The process also helps the family to develop a relationship with the clinician based on mutual understanding and cooperation.

In addition to the early stage, the typology and model of fluctuating family relationships are useful in the middle and late phases. Understanding the illness trajectory retrospectively will permit individualized case plans to be formulated, based on the individual characteristics and family experiences.

An example of potential clinical use of the FIS model would be in terms of the concept of expressed emotion (EE). Highly critical and hostile statements of family members have been shown to be predictive of relapse. Some authors have been critical of the concept of EE, hypothesizing that it is a bi-directional process, i.e., living with a person diagnosed with schizophrenia may result in family attitudes that are critical and hostile, and that in return, the attitudes affect the course of illness in a negative way. Application of the FIS model would pose an interesting set of questions that have not previously been addressed: What was the developmental phase of the high EE families? Was the onset of illness at a particularly out-of-phase point for the individual and the family? Which family members were required to alter their developmental course to the greatest degree? Are there other chronic conditions in the family that compound the effects of the new onset?

Identification of family cycles and individual developmental phases would help to pinpoint those families at greatest risk. An intervention goal of remaining at a distance from family may not be appropriate for patients at different developmental phases, and may need to be adapted. The intensity of the high EE interactions may be correlated with an out-of-cycle illness interacting with family and individual developmental stages.

Another clinical application of the comprehensive, developmental approach of the FIS model would be with psychoeducational interventions, noted by Rolland (1994). The developmental aspects of the individual and family should be incorporated into a psychoeducational treatment model to provide for the most effective and individualized care. The psychosocial improvement seen in later stages of schizophrenia by long-term follow-up studies may be related to a family and individual phase coinciding with the natural course of illness, which tends to plateau after the first five to ten years. Psychoeducational modules could be targeted toward specific time phases in the illness and focus on the family skills needed to confront particular psychosocial demands.

CONCLUSION

Clinical and research needs indicate the necessity of more accurate descriptions of the heterogeneous nature of the course of schizophrenia, in addition to developing and testing an integrated theoretical model that acknowledges the importance of the family. A longitudinal perspective will help to identify biological, social, and psychological changes that may influence intervention strategies.

The Family Involvement and Schizophrenia (FIS) model offers a method for the conceptualization and testing of the complex interaction of the individual, family, and illness developmental paths over the life cycle. The typology of illness includes the categories that are hypothesized to be most relevant to understanding the psychosocial aspects of schizophrenia, as well as providing a basis for cross-study comparisons. The time phases represent the changing developmental tasks and psychosocial demands for the individual and family.

Life cycle concepts of the individual and family developmental processes as integrated in the FIS highlight the periods of increased vulnerability to stress. Little is known about the interaction patterns between the family and the individual diagnosed with schizophrenia beyond early adulthood, and use of the typology, combined with continued gathering of family data as to their developmental stage, would facilitate the inclusion of the family in treatment planning in middle and late phases. Exploration of the changing developmental needs and demands of the illness, combined with those of the individual and family, may lead to an increase in interventions beyond the crisis stage. Periodic re-evaluations to assess strengths, weaknesses, and approaching transitions would facilitate an ongoing therapeutic connection, and would enable the clinician to address the life-long coping process.

REFERENCES

American Psychiatric Association (1987). *Diagnostic and statistical manual (DSM-IIIR).* Washington, D.C.: American Psychiatric Association Press.

Anderson, C., Hogarty, G., & Reiss, D. (1980). Family treatment of adult schizophrenia patients: A psychoeducational approach. *Schizophrenia Bulletin, 6* (3), 490-505.

Anderson, C., Reiss, D., & Hogarty, G. (1986). *Schizophrenia and the family.* New York: Gilford Press.

Anthony, W., & Liberman, R. (1986). The practice of psychiatric rehabilitation: Historical, conceptual, and research base. *Schizophrenia Bulletin, 12,* 542-559.

Attkisson, C., Cook, J., Karno, M., Lehman, A., McGlashan, T., Meltzer, H., O'Connor, M., Richardson, D., Rosenblatt, A., Wells, K., & Williams, J. (1992). Clinical services research. *Schizophrenia Bulletin, 18* (4), 561-626.

Bardenstein, K., McGlashan, T. (1990). Gender differences in affective, schizoaffective, and schizophrenic disorders: A review. *Schizophrenia Research, 3,* 159-192.

Barrowclough, C., & Tarrier, N. (1990). Social functioning in schizophrenic patients. The effects of expressed emotion and family intervention. *Social Psychiatry and Psychiatric Epidemiology, 25,* 125-130.

Beavers, W., & Voeller, M. (1983). Family models: Comparing and contrasting the Olson circumplex model with the Beavers systems model. *Family Process, 22,* 85-99.

Belitsky, R., & McGlashan, T.H. (1993). The manifestations of schizophrenia in late life: A dearth of data. *Schizophrenia Bulletin, 19* (4), 683-685.

Bernheim, K.F. (1990). Principles of professional and family collaboration. *Hospital and Community Psychiatry, 41* (12), 1353-1355

Bleuler, E. (1978). *The Schizophrenic disorders: The long-term patient and family studies.* Translated by Clemens, S.M., New Haven, Connecticut: Yale University Press.

Brown, G., Birley, J., & Wing, J. (1972). Influence of family life on the course of schizophrenic disorders: A replication. *British Journal of Psychiatry, 121,* 241-258.

Bulger, M.W., Wandersman, A., & Goldman, C.R. (1993). Burdens and gratifications of caregiving: Appraisal of parental care of adults with schizophrenia. *American Journal of Orthopsychiatry, 63* (2), 225-265.

Carpenter, W.T., Jr., & Kirkpatrick, B. (1988). The heterogeneity of the long-term course of schizophrenia. *Schizophrenia Bulletin, 14* (4), 645-652.

Carpenter, W.T., Kirkpatrick, B., & Buchanan, R.W. (1990). Conceptual approaches to the study of schizophrenia. In A. Kales, C.N. Stefanis, & J.A. Talbott (Eds.), *Recent advances in schizophrenia,* (pp. 93-113). New York: Springer-Verlag.

Ciompi, L. (1980). Catamnestic long-term study on the course of life and aging of schizophrenics. *Schizophrenia Bulletin, 6,* 606-618.

Ciompi, L. (1987). Review of follow-up studies on long-term evolution and aging in schizophrenia. In N.E. Miller, & G.D. Cohen (Eds.), *Schizophrenia and aging* (pp. 37-51). New York: Guilford Press.

Ciompi, L. (1988). *The psyche and schizophrenia.* Cambridge, MA: Harvard University Press.

Ciompi, L. (1989). The dynamics of complex biological-psychosocial systems: Four fundamental psychobiological mediators in the long-term evolution of schizophrenia. *British Journal of Psychiatry, 155 (Suppl. 5),* 15-21.

Combrinck-Graham, L. (1985). A developmental model for family systems. *Family Process, 24,* 139-150.

DeLisi, L.E. (1992). The significance of age of onset for schizophrenia. *Schizophrenia Bulletin, 18* (2), 209-215.

Falloon, I., Boyd, J., & McGill, C. (1984). *Family care of schizophrenia.* New York: Guilford Press.

Fromm-Reichman, F. (1950). *Principles of intensive psychotherapy.* Chicago: University of Chicago Press.

Goldstein, M.J. (1984). Family intervention programs. In A. Bellack (Ed.), *Schizophrenia: Treatment, management and rehabilitation.* New York: Grune & Stratton.

Goldstein, M.J. (1990). Psychosocial factors relating to etiology and course of schizophrenia. In M.I. Herz, S.J. Keith, & J.P. Docherty (Eds.), *Handbook of schizophrenia, Vol. 4: Psychosocial treatment of schizophrenia* (pp. 1-23). Amsterdam: Elsevier.

Goldstein, M.J., Rodnick, E.H., Evans, J.R., May, P.R., & Steinberg, M.R. (1978). Drug and family therapy in the aftercare treatment of acute schizophrenia. *Archives of General Psychiatry, 35,* 169-177.

Group for the Advancement of Psychiatry (GAP) (1992). *Beyond symptom suppression: Improving long-term outcomes of schizophrenia (Report No.134).* Washington, D.C.: American Psychiatric Press.

Heinrichs, D.W., Hanlon, T.E., & Carpenter, W.T. (1984). The Quality of Life Scale: An instrument for rating the schizophrenic deficit syndrome. *Schizophrenia Bulletin, 10,* 388-398.

Hogarty, G., Anderson, C., Reiss, D., Kornblith, S., Greenwald, D., Javna, C., & Madonia, M. (1986). Family psychoeducation, social skills training, and maintenance chemotherapy in the aftercare treatment of schizophrenia: I. One-year effects of a controlled study on relapse and expressed emotion. *Archives of General Psychiatry, 43,* 633-642.

Hogarty, G., Anderson, C., Reiss, D., Kornblith, S., Greenwald, D., Ulrich, R., and Carter, M. (1991). Family psychoeducation, social skills training and maintenance chemotherapy in the aftercare treatment of schizophrenia: II. Two-year effects of a controlled study on relapse and adjustment. *Archives of General Psychiatry, 48,* 340-347.

Krausz, M., & Muller-Thomsen, T. (1993). Schizophrenia with onset in adolescence: An 11-year follow-up. *Schizophrenia Bulletin, 19* (4), 831-841.

Leff, J., Kuipers, L., Berkowitz, R., & Sturgeon, D. (1982). A controlled trial of social intervention in the families of schizophrenic patients. *British Journal of Psychiatry, 141,* 121-134.

Leff, J. Kuipers, L., Berkowitz, R., & Sturgeon, D. (1985). A controlled trial of social intervention in the families of schizophrenic patients: Two-year follow-up. *British Journal of Psychiatry, 146,* 594-600.

Lefley, H.P. (1989). Family burden and family stigma in major illness. *American Psychologist 44* (3), 556-560.

Leventhal, D.B., Schuck, J.R., & Rothstein, H. (1984). Gender differences in schizophrenia. *Journal of Nervous and Mental Diseases, 172,* 464-467.

Levinson, D.J. (1978). *The seasons of a man's life.* New York: Guilford Press.

Levinson, D.J. (1986). A conception of adult development. *American Psychologist, 41,* 3-13.

Lidz, R., & Lidz, T. (1949). The family environment of schizophrenia patients. *American Journal of Psychiatry, 106,* 332-345.

Lin, K., & Kleinman, A.M. (1988). Psychopathology and clinical course of schizophrenia: A cross-cultural perspective. *Schizophrenia Bulletin, 14* (4), 555-568.

McFarlane, W., Dunne, E., Lukens, E., Newhart, M., McLaughlin-Toran, J., Deakins, S., & Horan, B. (1993). From research to clinical practice: Dissemination of New York State's family psychoeducational project. *Hospital and Community Pyschiatry, 44,* 265-270.

McGlashan, T.H., & Carpenter, W.T. (1988). Long-term follow-up studies of schizophrenia. *Schizophrenia Bulletin, 14,* (4) 497-500.

Marengo, J. (1994). Classifying the courses of schizophrenia. *Schizophrenia Bulletin, 20* (3), 519-536.

National Institute of Mental Health (1991). *Caring for people with severe mental disorders.* (DHHS Publication No. ADM 91-1762). Washington, DC: U.S. Government Printing Office.

Nicholson, I., & Neufeld, R. (1992). A dynamic vulnerability perspective on stress and schizophrenia. *American Journal of Orthopsychiatry, 62,* 117-130.

Nuechterlein, K.H. (1987). Vulnerability models: State of the art. In H. Hafner, W. Gattaz, & W. Jangerik (Eds.). *Searches for the cause of schizophrenia.* Berlin: Springer-Verlag.

Nuechterlein, K.H., & Dawson, M.E. (1984). A heuristic vulnerability/stress model of schizophrenia episodes. *Schizophrenia Bulletin, 10* (2), 300-312.

Pepper, B., & Ryglewicz, H. (Eds.). (1984). *Advances in treating the young adult chronic patient* (New Directions in Mental Health Services, no. 212). San Francisco: Jossey-Bass.

Rolland, J.S. (1994). *Families, illness, and disability.* New York: Basic Books.

Salonkongas, K. (1983). Prognostic implications of the sex of schizophrenic patients. *British Journal of Psychiatry, 142,* 145-151.

Seeman, M.V. (1986). Current outcome in schizophrenia: Women vs. men. *Acta Psychiatrica Scandinavia, 73,* 609-617.

Straube, E., & Oades, R. (Eds.). (1992). *Schizophrenia: Empirical research and findings.* New York: Academic Press.

Strauss, J. (1989). Mediating processes in schizophrenia–Toward a new dynamic psychiatry. *British Journal of Psychiatry, 155* (Suppl. 5), 22-28.

Talbott, J.A. (1990). Current perspectives in the United States on the chronically mentally ill. In A. Kales, C. Stefanis, & J. Talbot (Eds.), *Recent advances in schizophrenia* (pp. 279-295). New York: Springer-Verlag.

Vaughn, C., & Leff, J. (1976). The influence of family and social factors on the course of psychiatric illness. *British Journal of Psychiatry, 129,* 125-137.

Wynne, L.C. (1988). The natural histories of schizophrenia processes. *Schizophrenia Bulletin, 14* (4), 653-659.

Yank, G.R., Bentley, K.J., Hargrove, D.S. (1993). The vulnerability-stress model of schizophrenia: Advances in psychosocial treatment. *American Journal of Orthopsychiatry, 63* (1), 55-69.

Yassa, R., & Suranyi-Cadotte, B. (1993). Clinical characteristics of late-onset schizophrenia and delusional disorder. *Schizophrenia Bulletin, 19* (4), 701-707.

Zubin, J., & Spring, B. (1977). Vulnerability: A new view of schizophrenia. *Journal of Abnormal Psychology, 86* (2), 103-126.

The Role of the Family
in Promoting Drug Free Communities
in Nigeria

Isidore S. Obot, PhD, MPH

SUMMARY. Drug abuse and its consequences have become an additional source of concern for the survival of the African family and, in particular, Nigerian families. The focus of this paper is on the relevance of the Nigerian family in the prevention of drug and alcohol related problems. This paper discusses the ways in which the Nigerian family can serve as an effective resource in helping to control the spread of alcohol and drug abuse and the problems associated with drugs in the community. *[Article copies available for a fee from The Haworth Document Delivery Service: 1-800-342-9678. E-mail address: <getinfo@haworthpressinc.com> Website: <http://www.HaworthPress.com> © 2001 by The Haworth Press, Inc. All rights reserved.]*

KEYWORDS. Nigeria, Africa, family, drugs, prevention and treatment

---

Isidore S. Obot is affiliated with the Department of Psychology, University of Jos, Jos, Nigeria.

Address correspondence to: Isidore S. Obot, PhD, MPH, Centre for Research and Information on Substance Abuse, Box 10331, University Post Office, Jos, Nigeria (E-mail: isobot@hisen.org or isobot@yahoo.com).

An earlier version of this paper was presented at the XVI World Conference of Therapeutic Communities, Kuala Lumpur, Malaysia, September 1993.

[Haworth co-indexing entry note]: "The Role of the Family in Promoting Drug Free Communities in Nigeria." Obot, Isidore S. Co-published simultaneously in *Journal of Family Social Work* (The Haworth Social Work Practice Press, an imprint of The Haworth Press, Inc.) Vol. 6, No. 1, 2001, pp. 53-67; and: *Families and Health: Cross-Cultural Perspectives* (ed: Jorge Delva) The Haworth Social Work Practice Press, an imprint of The Haworth Press, Inc., 2001, pp. 53-67. Single or multiple copies of this article are available for a fee from The Haworth Document Delivery Service [1-800-342-9678, 9:00 a.m. - 5:00 p.m. (EST). E-mail address: getinfo@haworthpressinc.com].

53

INTRODUCTION

Compared to other parts of the world, health and economic indicators of development in African countries are abysmally low. In particular, infant and child mortality rates, life expectancy, literacy rate, and GNP per capita have not shown any appreciable improvement and have, in fact, declined in some cases. Though many countries have implemented policies that promise greater availability of preventive health care and literacy programs, the worsening economic situation in the continent and rapid population growth have made these programs less effective.

While the problem of diseases has been around for many years, the African family is now faced with another set of serious problems. Almost every country on the continent is experiencing an increase in alcohol and other drug-related problems, and in HIV/AIDS cases. Drug related psychiatric morbidity, family disruption, violence, and accidents have all been on the rise. The arrival of new drugs—cocaine and heroin—in the youth drug scene, together with the increasing availability of alcohol and tobacco, and the rising incidence of self medication with dangerous pharmaceuticals, have brought a sense of urgency to the situation. Drug abuse and its consequences have become an additional source of concern for the survival of the African family and in particular among Nigerian families. The focus of this paper is on the relevance of the Nigerian family in the prevention of drug and alcohol related problems. This paper discusses the ways in which families in Nigeria can serve as an effective resource in helping to control the spread of alcohol and drug abuse and the problems associated with drugs in the community.

THE PREVALENCE OF SUBSTANCE ABUSE IN NIGERIA

Alcohol is one of the oldest drugs used by Africans. In its traditional (local) forms, (e.g., palm wine, *burukutu, pito*) the substance plays a vital role in African social life—in marriages, negotiations, and the appeasement of the gods. In these culturally defined situations alcohol is consumed by adults or by children under the watchful eyes of their parents. Thus, instances of intoxication are rare and meet with strong disapproval. These traditional beverages are still available today, but there has also been a large increase in the production of commercial beer, wine and spirits. For example, there were four breweries in Nigeria in 1977, but there are approximately 40 today, producing a large number of brands of beer and stout. In addition, since the ban on the importation of beer was lifted a few years ago, the Nigerian marketplace is now filled with a wide variety of European brands.

Population surveys reveal that consumption of alcoholic drinks, especially beer, has kept pace with production. In a survey of heads of household, 52% of the respondents described themselves as drinkers with one third of the drinkers consuming 1.8 litres of beer per day on the average (Obot, 1993a). Alcohol consumption among the youth population is widespread and frequent intoxication has been reported in some student groups. Yet, the link between alcohol, health and social problems in Nigeria and other African countries has not received much attention, even though the high rates of accidents and psychiatric morbidity have been associated with excessive consumption of alcohol (International Council on Alcohol and Addictions, 1988).

The use of other substances has been a source of concern in Nigeria and other African countries for many years. In the early 1960s, less than 20 years after the plant started growing in Nigeria, Cannabis use became a problem among Nigerian urban youth. Reports from psychiatric hospitals showed that high proportions of young people admitted into hospitals in the Lagos area had histories of cannabis abuse (Asuni, 1964; Lambo, 1965). More recent available data indicate that cannabis accounts for up to 8% of all cases, 60% of drug-related cases in psychiatric hospitals (Obot & Olaniyi, 1991), and nearly 16% of casualty cases (ICAA, 1988). Cannabis is also the drug most often used in combination with other drugs, especially alcohol and cocaine. A survey of students showed that up to 20% had tried cannabis at least once in their lives (ICAA, 1988).

In the middle 1980s, cocaine and heroin became a part of the Nigerian drug scene. The drugs were originally smuggled through Nigerian airports to North America and Western Europe. Not long after, young people in large Nigerian cities were exposed to these drugs and started using them. The effect has been traumatic. For example, in a recent study of admissions into four psychiatric hospitals from 1984-1988, cocaine- and heroin-related cases showed a rapid increase in the five-year period, from one case in 1984 to dozens in 1988 (Obot & Olaniyi, 1991). A study of the general population has shown that 0.8% and 0.2% of the respondents had "ever used" cocaine and heroin, respectively (ICAA, 1988). The recent introduction of crack cocaine into the country will only add to Nigeria's drug related problems. Most Nigerian users of cocaine and heroin smoke these drugs, but there is evidence that injecting drug use is becoming the preferred mode of use among some youth groups in large cities (Adelekan, 2000).

Cigarette smoking also is a problem in many African countries. In Nigeria, up to 22% of the adult population describe themselves as regular smokers and a high proportion of them smoke at least half a pack of cigarettes a day (Obot, 1990). Among male students in secondary and post-secondary schools about 29% smoke cigarettes.

Tranquilizers (e.g., valium) and analgesics (e.g., paracetamol) are used extensively by adults without prescription. The increasing use of these sleeping aids and pain relievers may be connected with the harsh realities of modern family life in Nigeria. This problem is compounded by parents who depend to a great extent on unregistered drug stores which provide an assortment of pharmaceuticals that are often placebos, expired or diluted. There have been many reports of children who have died because they were given contaminated or expired analgesics.

The abuse of stimulants by students as well as drivers trying to stay awake also has been reported. Students use amphetamines or "brain pills" for energy and wakefulness especially during examination periods. Drivers on long journeys chew kolanuts or use any of a number of stimulant drugs for similar reasons.

The use of inhalants (e.g., petrol, glue, kerosene) is also on the rise. In Lagos, 35% of the secondary students interviewed in a study by the International Council on Alcohol and Addictions (ICAA, 1988) reported using an inhalant at least once. A survey of secondary school students in northern Nigeria showed that the prevalence of lifetime use of organic solvents was 25.7% and use in the past month of was 11.2% (Obot, 1993b).

THE NIGERIAN FAMILY

The Structure and Dynamics of the Nigerian Family

Whenever children or their parents abuse alcohol or other types of drugs the effect is felt in the entire family. But the family can also be the direct or indirect cause of drug abuse because what goes on in the family often contributes to the initiation of drug use by children. This realization has made the study of family dynamics in drug abuse an active area of research interest. What are the characteristics of the Nigerian family that are relevant to an understanding of the drug problem? In what ways can family dynamics serve as a help or hindrance in drug abuse initiation, maintenance, and treatment? The rest of this paper will be devoted to answering these questions.

There is no single profile of the family across all groups in Nigeria, but there are several areas of similarity in terms of family structure. Most Nigerian families have been exposed to those influences which have affected the dynamics of family life in modern Africa. Yet, while many changes have taken place, there has been resilience in several areas. These are discussed next.

The African family is large in size. Families in traditional Nigeria tend to be large and inclusive. The size of the family is influenced by at least two factors:

a. The number of children: Even among transitional and modern Africans the perception is still strong that the family is better off with more children. The average number of children per family in most African countries is more than five.

b. Polygamy (in particular polygyny): The number of African men who are married to more than one wife is still high, in spite of western influences. Because a high proportion of Africans are Muslim, marrying more than one wife is an acceptable practice.

The family is inclusive or extended. This is the most often discussed feature of the African family. The extended family structure is different from the nuclear family in that it includes grandparents, uncles, aunts, cousins and siblings in a loose or tight network of relationships. The value of the extended family lies in the interdependence that it engenders and also in that it provides multiple caregivers for children. The children are exposed to the direct influences of at least three generations in the family and receive the attention of parents and other relatives living in the same compound. According to Esen (1973), the extended family structure provides the child greater opportunity for identification, a large variety of role models, the availability of someone to turn to at anytime, and the opportunity to develop a positive attitude toward asking for and receiving help.

There is a clear sense of hierarchy and elders are respected. The father is the direct head of the household. Children must obey him, respect those who are older than them in the extended family, and be at the service of their relatives.

Loyalty to the family and clan is expected. The family is part of a network of families that constitutes the clan. Loyalty to the clan is a family virtue and expected because the clan is the source of identity. A traditional saying that highlights this value is: "I am because we are; because we are, therefore I am." This saying describes the relationship of the individual to the family and his or her clan. One implication of loyalty is that conformity is expected and individualism is discouraged.

Children are socialized to receive and give care. Of particular relevance to the building of drug free communities is the role of the family as caregiver (Esen, 1973). Care is central to the African way of life; the African is his brother's keeper. As the African child is socialized, s/he is trained to give and accept care as a matter of course. Through close contact and language the child receives "the comfort of care from others" and "soon learns to expect it at appropriate times and to give it to those needing it" (Esen, 1973, p. 7). Through the extended family structure the child receives care not only from parents but also from grandparents, cousins, uncles and aunts, and siblings living within the same environment. The child is expected to learn from these relatives "not only the roles appropriate to his sex, but also ways of feeling and communicating those feelings as he develops from stage to stage" (Esen, 1973, p. 11). Because children are highly valued, there can never be too many. They are regarded as a gift from God, a link to the past and a bridge to the future.

THE FAMILY IN A CHANGING SOCIETY

In recent years a number of changes have occurred that have affected the structure and well being of the Nigerian family as described above. These changes can be found in different areas of Nigerian life and culture.

a. A high level of rural-urban migration has reduced the significance of the extended family and encouraged the growth of nuclear families. Uncles, aunts, grandparents and cousins have lost much of their influence in bringing up children. This burden has fallen on the parents, hired help, and other resources that the city can provide. But life in the city is not as stable as life in a small village community where everybody is in some way related. The city, especially for a new arrival, is a stressful environment with a direct affect on the family.

b. Increasing rates of divorce, teenage pregnancy, and untimely deaths of spouses from accidents, "diseases of civilization" (e.g., heart disease, cancer, alcoholism), and HIV/AIDS have combined to produce many single-parent families.

b. There has been an increasing number of orphaned children either because the children are abandoned at birth or because of high rates of maternal mortality, especially among young unmarried women.

c. More parents are absent from home for extended periods of time for economic reasons. For example, there are more and more cases in which the father lives and works in the city while the mother lives with the children in the village. But more significant is the fact that both parents are now often absent from the home in families where the wife and husband have modern jobs. Because of the increased educational achievement of women, more of them are participating in the workplace. This implies that more children are being taken care of by baby-sitters who are often unqualified to carry out their duties. The care that the African child now receives is minimal or, in some cases, nonexistent.

e. Children are experiencing increased trauma at a young age due to battering, sexual abuse, and neglect. The exploitation of children for economic reasons is also seen in the use of children for street trading and early marriage for the purpose of taking bride wealth.

d. Life in urban areas also encourages individualism and less identification with traditional groups. Urban children identify more with peers than with authority figures, including parents and grandparents. The result of this may be intergenerational conflicts among family members. Instead of seeing themselves as the small links in a long chain, children define themselves as different from adults, and thus separate from them. Rebellion may occur in many ways, including the use and abuse of drugs. The traditional socialization of the African child is geared towards conformity with the norms of the clan and the larger society, and there is no room for rebellion.

FAMILY AND EARLY CHILDHOOD FACTORS IN DRUG ABUSE

Concerns about the way family dynamics affect or influence drug-using behaviors of children has received increased attention of researchers and prevention experts in recent years. Kumpfer and Alvarado (1995) describe a number of risk factors to explain drug abuse that include individual, family, peer, and community characteristics. Factors related to drug use found in Western countries and in Nigeria are:

1. Parental and sibling use of alcohol and drugs: As mentioned earlier, this is an important variable in the initiation of drug use among children. For example, male children of parents with alcohol problems are many times more likely to develop alcohol problems than other children (Jennison & Johnson, 1998; Obot, Wagner, & Anthony, 2000). How much of this is the result of genetic predisposition or modeling is not clear.

2. Inadequate socialization: Poor socialization of the child may result in weak bonds with parents and/or significant persons in the social environment and a strong attachment to delinquent peers. One consequence of this is the development of problem behaviors including drug abuse. In a tripartite model of African socialization of the substance abuser Peltzer (1989), provides some evidence that major crises in authority, group, and body-mind-environment dimensions are responsible for the initiation of drug use.

3. Marital discord: Discord between husband and wife is a risk factor for psychological disorders because discord leads to family disorganization. The problem behavior of the child is often an attempt to reunite the parents by focusing them on his or her problem. Research has also shown that when the family is not cohesive parent-child attachment and warmth will be lacking (National Institute on Drug Abuse [NIDA], 1987). The children may grow up with low self-esteem and generally poor emotional well being and therefore may use drugs to "feel good." In a family where one parent is distant and the other is indulgent and over-protective, the condition is set for the beginning of problem behaviors including drug abuse. In Nigeria, Ebigbo (1989) has shown how psychopathology develops in children because of conflicts between parents. According to this author, treatment is dependent on the resolution of the conflict in a family therapy setting.

4. Family norms and attitudes: Norms and attitudes which do not disapprove of drugs and alcohol encourage their use. A general population survey of alcohol use in Nigeria showed that adults are generally very disapproving of the use of alcohol by young people either at home, with friends, or at social functions (Obot, 1993a).

5. Stress in the family: Crises within the family can precipitate drug use or any other form of abnormal behavior as a way of coping with the stress brought by the crises. Ebigbo (1989) has also shown that the factors associated with psychological disturbance among Nigerian students include: coming from a family with more than five children,

coming from a polygamous home, being the last born child, and having a poor father.

IMPACT OF DRUG ABUSE ON THE FAMILY

Interest in the role of drugs in family functioning is necessitated by the observed negative consequences. Commenting on the hazard of alcohol abuse in Southern Africa, Smith (1982) stated that:

> The tendency for the very poor and the privileged to be particularly affected has serious consequences. For the very poor, who live on the edge of survival, an alcoholic father may mean death for members of the family. Furthermore, alcoholism and malnutrition are a particularly unhappy and dangerous combination. The society is likely to suffer badly if the professionals and technocrats are removed through alcohol problems. (p. 248)

The death of the breadwinner is the most serious consequence of alcohol and other drug abuse on the family. But there are other ways in which drug use can affect the family either directly or indirectly.

1. A drug-abusing parent may abuse the children or spouse physically.
2. Addicted parents are prone to neglect the educational and social needs of their children.
3. A family with a drug abuser is likely to be unstable and prone to more conflict than might have been the case without the problem.
4. Children of drug abusing parents are predisposed to becoming drug abusers themselves.

THE ROLE OF THE FAMILY IN PREVENTION AND TREATMENT OF ALCOHOL AND DRUG PROBLEMS

The essence of this paper is that the family is implicated in the initiation and maintenance of drug abuse behaviors. Therefore to control the problem the family (not just the parents or children but the whole system as a unit) must be actively involved. The role of the family in alcohol and other drug abuse initiation, prevention and treatment lies in family system theory. The basic assumption of this theory is that significant persons in the family influence the way members relate to each other and also influence the onset or solution of the problem. In treatment, familial influences may facilitate the intervention because there can be a large number of persons available who can assist the person addicted to substances.

While it is true that the Nigerian family has changed in recent years as a result of external influences, the extended family structure has been generally resilient enough to continue to play the role of a control and social support system in the prevention and treatment of drug abuse. The implication seems to be that if the family, whether nuclear or extended, is strong and united the problem of drug abuse will not arise and if it does will be resolved successfully.

One way that parents can prevent drug abuse in children is through the example of abstinence from drugs and regulated use of alcohol. Even the use of prescription drugs (generally purchased without prescription in Nigeria) should be done in such a way that children do not grow up believing drugs are the cure for all ills, whether physical or psychological. Apart from good example, it is important for parents and other members of the extended family to be involved actively in the education of the children by showing interest in their work. Poor performance in school is associated with drug abuse and vice versa, hence the effect of parent involvement may be improved academic performance and reduced chances of drug use. The extended family structure makes it possible to assign specific roles to competent individuals when parents are not capable or available. When the extended family is effective, early recognition of a problem is also possible. Recognizing the early warning signs of substance abuse and taking appropriate action can help to prevent the problem from getting out of control.

In the early stages of life the family is, of course, responsible for the socialization of the child. This process of introducing the child to the ways of the group is a community affair. All members of the extended family in the family compound and other members of the clan carry it out. Morals and norms are taught using different methods. Folklore is important, so also is imitation and practical training. This approach can be adapted specifically to the prevention of drug abuse in the community and, in fact, the operation of a therapeutic community. In the treatment and rehabilitation of an addicted member the role of the family as a unit becomes critical. Drug abuse is a chronic, relapsing disorder. From the beginning of treatment to long-term rehabilitation, social support is required. Especially in situations where there are few social services for recovering addicts (as is the case in most African countries), only the family can guarantee such support.

Traditionally the Nigerian family is involved in all aspects of substance abuse treatment. It is often the case that even estranged members of the family are brought together in the process of seeking help for a troubled relative. Depending on skills or acquired status in the family, a member is assigned specific roles in the "therapy managing group." Such roles include:

- Deciding on the type of therapy (western, traditional, spiritual, or a combination of these)
- Looking for and consulting the healer
- Paying for treatment
- Attending meetings called by the healer
- Deciding on post-treatment rehabilitation

Demonstration of family unity is important in therapeutic interventions. When members of the family are summoned by the healer to a meeting it is often because the healer traces the source of the problem to a jealous family member (Ebigbo, 1989). When a family member takes great pain to be present at such a meeting it is not always for the sake of the sick member but also to avoid those present from talking about the absent person (Ebigbo, 1989). This implied declaration of innocence is important in polygamous situations where the source of the problem can easily be attributed to a co-wife or a distant cousin.

The Family in Treatment: The Aro Experience

The family model of the Aro Neuropsychiatric Hospital in Nigeria has shown that the participation of a member of the family in some aspects of treatment is beneficial. The Aro Hospital village system started in the 1950s. The hospital is named after the village where it is situated on the outskirts of Abeokuta, a small town in Western Nigeria. According to this model, a relative is expected to live with the patient in order to take care of his/her personal needs, take the patient to the hospital from the village, and attend social activities with the patient (Jegede, 1982). Every attempt is made to recreate the village environment familiar to the patient. The community in which the village system is located is expected to participate in the planning and execution of the programs. The central feature of the system is the participation of relatives in the treatment process. Because of the extended family structure and what

Esen (1973) calls the African "care syndrome," there is always a relative willing or able to assist the individual when attending treatment.

Family support has been shown to be an important factor in treatment success (Carise, 2000) in other parts of the world. That is why organized family groups (e.g., Al-Anon) have become an essential component of treatment in many countries. While there are few of these organizations in African countries today, they will become necessary for the rehabilitation of drug dependent persons as the African society becomes more urban and traditional group structures become weaker.

While the family is certainly a positive force in prevention and treatment, it can also serve as a hindrance. When, for example, a family has rigid boundaries, the tendency is to keep out potential help and seek to solve the problem itself. Sometimes this is because the family trusts its ability to handle the problem but often it is an attempt to conceal what may be regarded as embarrassing to the family. By becoming over-involved with the troubled member and failing to release him or her for external care, the family ends up as a negative influence in recovery. In polygamous families, suspicions and conflicts among children of different mothers can also be detrimental to the recovery of a disturbed member.

STRENGTHENING THE NIGERIAN FAMILY TO WORK TOWARDS BUILDING OF DRUG FREE COMMUNITIES

The family cannot be expected to carry out its functions in isolation. The reality of life in Nigeria today is that the family is under stress and needs help to cope with difficult socio-economic conditions. Some of the resources needed in a changing society can only be provided centrally through social policies that are aimed at manipulating the environment. Many researchers such as Kayongo-Male and Onyango (1984), have discussed the areas that need to be addressed. Some of these areas are directly related to the control of drug abuse. All of them, together with the inherent characteristics of African societies (e.g., the care syndrome), are important in building healthy communities in a modern society. They include:

Health Care

- Pre-and post-natal care.
- The establishment of more facilities for treatment and rehabilitation of drug dependent persons.

- Family planning services to help prevent risky pregnancies and therefore reduce the incidence of maternal death and the birth of children who may grow up to become problem children.

Education

- Making formal education more accessible to women.
- Conducting literacy classes for adults.
- Teaching parenting skills to urban mothers because of increasing confusion about how to raise children (especially regarding the best approaches to discipline children) in a modern society where there are conflicts between old and new ways.
- Making available and accessible information on drugs, drug abuse prevention and treatment and where to seek for help when needed.

Social Welfare Programs

- Day care for children.
- School lunch programs.
- Recreational and other social opportunities for children.
- Counseling services, especially in the cities because traditional support is weak or sometimes unavailable.

Legal Protection for Women and Children

- Legislating against child and forced marriages.
- Giving equal rights to women in marriage and divorce.
- Controlling child labor and other forms of child abuse.

Added to these, there is a need for the provision of factual and clear information about drugs and drug abuse to families in both rural and urban areas. For example, many parents are not aware of the drug behaviors of their children and are often at a loss as to what do when they discover that their children are using drugs (Obot, 2000). In many communities, alcoholism is not regarded as a serious problem and, therefore, help is not given when it would be useful. A sustained community education program using a network of community health workers and drug abuse control agencies, including NGOs, is an essential feature in any effort to promote drug free lifestyles. In Jos, Nigeria, the Center for Research and Information on Substance Abuse (CRISA), a private non-profit community service organization, was set up for this purpose and is slowly achieving its objectives.

CONCLUSION

In conclusion, it is important to emphasize the need to maintain the central role of women in the African family. Unfortunately, this primary caregiver suffers from neglect and has to fight for her rights (Imam, Pittin, & Omole, 1989). There is an urgent need for improvements in the legal status of women and other areas listed above if the African family will continue to play a vital role in preventing and eradicating social problems in a fast changing society. Unhappy, hungry and traumatized families cannot be expected to perform these functions effectively. What will save the modern Nigerian family are the implementation of human-centered social policies which do not focus on limited parameters of economic development, along with the maintenance and refinement of those old ways which have made the Nigerian family a veritable institution of care in the community. In substance abuse as in other social problems prevention is indeed better than cure. The most effective vehicles for prevention and, indeed, treatment are strong, healthy and loving families.

REFERENCES

Adelekan, M. (2000). Injecting drug use among "area boys" in Nigeria. Personal communication.

Asuni, T. (1964). Sociopsychiatric problems of cannabis in Nigeria. *Bulletin on Narcotics, 16*(2), 17.

Carise, D. (2000). Effects of family involvement on length of stay and treatment completion rates with cocaine and alcohol abusers. In J. Delva (Ed.), *Substance abuse issues among families in diverse populations* (pp. 79-94). New York: The Haworth Press, Inc.

Ebigbo, P. (1989). The practice of family therapy in the University of Nigeria Teaching Hospital, Enugu. In K. Peltzer & P. O. Ebigbo (Eds.), *Clinical Psychology in Africa.* Enugu: Working Group for African Psychology.

Esen, A. (1973). *The care syndrome: A resource for counseling in Africa.* Paper presented at First African Regional Conference of the International Association of Cross-Cultural Psychology, Ibadan, Nigeria, 2-3 April.

Imam, A., Pittin, R., & Omole, H. (1989). *Women and the Family in Nigeria.* Dakar(Senegal): CODESRIA Book Series.

International Council on Alcohol and Addictions (1988). *Report of Research on Substance Abuse in some Urban and Rural Areas of Nigeria*. Lausanne: Author.

Jegede, R. O. (1982). Aro village system in perspective. In O. A. Erinosho & N. W. Bell (Eds.), *Mental Health in Africa*. Ibadan: Ibadan University Press.

Jennison, K.M., & Johnson, K.A. (1998). Alcohol dependence in adult children of alcoholics: Longitudinal evidence of early risk. *Journal of Drug Education, 28*(1), 19-37.

Kayongo-Male, D., & Onyango, P. (1984). *The Sociology of the African Family*. London: Longman.

Kumpfer, K.L., & Alvarado, R. (1995). Strengthening families to prevent drug use in multiethnic youth. In G. J. Botvin, S. Schinke, & M. A. Orlandi (Eds.), *Drug abuse prevention with multiethnic youth* (pp. 255-294). Thousand Oaks, CA: SAGE Pubs.

Lambo, T.A. (1965). Medical and social problems of drug addiction in West Africa. *The West African Medical Journal, 14*, 236-254.

National Institute on Drug Abuse (1987). *Drug Abuse and Drug Abuse Research: The Second Triennial Report to Congress*. DHHS Publication No.(ADM) 87-1486. Washington, DC., U.S. Government Printing Office.

Obot, I.S., & Olaniyi, A.A. (1991). Drug-induced psychiatric disorders in four Nigerian hospitals, 1984-1988. *Nigerian Journal of Psychology, 8*(1), 13-16.

Obot, I.S. (1993a). *Alcohol Behaviour and Attitudes in Nigeria: A General Population Survey in the Middlebelt*. Jos, Nigeria: Centre for Development Studies (Monograph Series).

Obot, I.S. (1993b). Epidemiology of inhalant abuse in Nigeria. In N. Kozel Z. Sloboda & M. de la Rosa (Eds.), *Epidemiology of Inhalant Abuse: An International Perspective*. NIDA Research Monograph 148. Rockville: National Institute on Drug Abuse.

Obot, I.S. (2000). Assessment of drug use among Nigerian secondary school students and the views of their parents. Lagos: United Nations International Drug Control Programme (in press).

Obot, I.S. (1990). The use of tobacco products among Nigerian adults: A general population survey. *Drug and Alcohol Dependence, 26*, 203-208.

Obot, I.S., Wagner, F.A., & Anthony, J.C. (2000). Early onset drug use among children of parents with alcohol problems: Data from a national epidemiologic survey. Manuscript under review.

Peltzer, K. ((1989). Psychosocial counselling of persons with substance-related disorders. In K. Peltzer & P. O. Ebigbo (Eds.), *Clinical Psychology in Africa*. Enugu: Working Group for African Psychology.

Smith, R. (1982). Alcohol in the third world: A chance to avoid a miserable trap. *British Medical Journal, 284*, 183-185.

A Study of Family Fighting
and Illegal Drug Use Among Adults
Who Completed
Substance Abuse Treatment

Scott Ryan, PhD
Jorge Delva, PhD
Samuel J. Gruber, MSW

SUMMARY. Violence and substance abuse within families has reached epidemic proportions in the United States. To help illuminate this issue, this study investigated the suspected association between family fighting and substance use taking into consideration individual, social and environmental factors. Estimates of the association between family fighting and illegal drug use were obtained using a convenience sample of 289 adults that completed substance abuse treatment in Florida. The data were collected via a Computerized Assisted Telephone Interview (CATI) method during the summer of 1999. Illegal drug use was positively associated with frequent family fighting (OR = 4.53; 95% CI =

Scott Ryan, Jorge Delva, and Samuel J. Gruber are affiliated with Florida State University.

Address correspondence to: Scott Ryan, School of Social Work, Florida State University, Tallahassee, FL 32306-2570.

This research was funded by the State of Florida Department of Children and Families.

The views presented in this manuscript are solely those of the authors and do not represent those of the Department.

[Haworth co-indexing entry note]: "A Study of Family Fighting and Illegal Drug Use Among Adults Who Completed Substance Abuse Treatment." Ryan. Scott. Jorge Delva, and Samuel J. Gruber. Co-published simultaneously in *Journal of Family Social Work* (The Haworth Social Work Practice Press, an imprint of The Haworth Press. Inc.) Vol. 6. No. 1. 2001. pp. 69-78: and: *Families and Health: Cross-Cultural Perspectives* (ed: Jorge Delva) The Haworth Social Work Practice Press, an imprint of The Haworth Press. Inc.. 2001. pp. 69-78. Single or multiple copies of this article are available for a fee from The Haworth Document Delivery Service [1-800-342-9678. 9:00 a.m. - 5:00 p.m. (EST). E-mail address: getinfo@haworthpressinc.com].

1.89-10.82) and inversely associated with social support (OR = .49; 95% CI = 1.00-1.13), even after adjustments for demographic and other social characteristics were considered. Practice implications include the need for integrated treatment services, interventions utilizing social support systems and aftercare services to ensure treatment adherence. *[Article copies available for a fee from The Haworth Document Delivery Service: 1-800-342-9678. E-mail address: <getinfo@haworthpressinc.com> Website: <http://www.HaworthPress.com> © 2001 by The Haworth Press, Inc. All rights reserved.]*

KEYWORDS. Treatment, drug use, family, violence

INTRODUCTION

This brief study reports the finding of an association found between family fighting and substance use among individuals that completed substance abuse treatment. Research has shown that illegal drug use and violence are highly correlated (Bureau of Justice Statistics, 1994; Gorney, 1989). Family violence is one such form of violence generally found to be correlated with alcohol and other drug use (Easton, Swan and Sinha, 2000; Holtzworth-Munroe & Stuart, 1994; Maiden, 1997). Research also has shown that family violence in the form of child abuse frequently occurs in families with substance abusers (Besinger, Garland, Litrownik & Landsverk, 1999; Black & Mayer, 1980; Corvo & Carpenter, 2000; Wolock & Magura, 1996). Stanton's work in the 1970s brought increased attention to the role substance abuse filled within the family context and interpersonal relationships under which individuals use drugs (Stanton, 1978, 1980). Maladaptive family functioning can hinder a person's recovery. However, it is important to indicate that we are not suggesting that families cause a family member to use drugs. Instead it is suggested that difficulties families encounter relating to one another in a healthy and supportive manner, serve as stressors that generate an environment conducive to maladaptive coping behaviors, of which drug use is one such behavior.

Reductions in family fighting, drug consumption, and drug related problems have been observed among individuals that complete substance abuse treatment (Delva, Allgood, Morrell, & McNeece, in press; Hubbard et al., 1989; Maiden, 1997; Substance Abuse and Mental Health Services Administration, 1998). As such, the importance of understanding the influences of families on the individual's recovery cannot be overemphasized if drug relapse and family violence are to be prevented (Benshoff & Janikowski, 2000; Friedman, 1998). In this cross-sectional study, we seek to answer the following question: Is the occurrence of illegal drug use among individuals that completed substance abuse treatment more common among those that report greater frequency of family fighting when compared to those that do not report family fighting?

METHOD

Participants and Procedures

The data used in this study were collected in 1999 via a Computer Assisted Telephone Interviewing (CATI) survey of 499 adults who received substance abuse treatment in the State of Florida in 1998-1999. In this study we analyze the data for the 289 participants who completed residential, outpatient, methadone, or other types of treatment.

Measures

A 10-minute CATI interview was conducted by a professional survey lab. The questionnaire included questions on the person's demographic characteristics (i.e., self-reported racial and ethnic background, marital status), mental health problems (i.e., symptoms of depression and anxiety), alcohol consumption and drug use six to twelve months after receiving substance abuse treatment, social support, frequency of family fighting, frequency of church attendance, neighborhood safety, among others. All research was conducted in accordance to federal regulations governing confidentiality of Alcohol and Drug Abuse client records, 42 Code of Federal Regulations Part 2.

Data Analysis

The characteristics of drug users and non-users were first compared using bivariate analysis. Subsequently, the data were analyzed using multiple logistic regression with the SPSS software. The odds ratios representing the association between frequency of family fighting and drug use were obtained after adjusting for selected demographic characteristics, social support, and church attendance.

RESULTS

Description of Participants

Table 1 displays the distribution of drug use across selected characteristics of the sample. A larger proportion of 18-25 year olds reported using drugs than older individuals. Similarly, there was a larger proportion of drug use among never married individuals when compared to married or other groups. Individuals who reported frequent family fighting, not having social support, and not attending church also were more likely to report drug use. No other significant bivariate association was observed.

Family Fighting and Drug Use

There was a significant association between frequency of family fighting and drug use, even after adjustments were made for the potential distorting influences of covariates such as age, marital status, availability of social support, and church attendance (see Table 2). Specifically, individuals who indicated they fought sometimes with their families in the month prior to the interview were 180% more likely than those that did not fight to have used drugs (Odds Ratio [OR] = 2.80; 95% Confidence Interval [CI] = 1.21-6.45). Those that experienced frequent fighting were 353% more likely to have used drugs than those that did report fighting with their families (OR = 4.53; 95%CI = 1.89-10.82). Also, individuals who indicated having someone they could count on in case of need were half as likely to have used drugs than those without social support (OR = 0.49; 95%CI = 1.00-1.13).

DISCUSSION

The data suggest a strong association between the frequency in which individuals argue with their families and drug use. Unfortunately, the cross-sectional nature of the design does not allow us to determine a temporal association between these variables. In addition, Friedman (1998), in a review of the literature, posits that if there is no control for the specific type of drug used, a washing out effect may impact the relationships of the drugs upon the family violence variable. The small sample size did not allow us to study the association between specific drugs and family fighting raising the possibility that important

TABLE 1. Distribution of Drug Use Across Sample Characteristics

Characteristic	Sample (N = 289)	Used Drugs n	%
Sex			
Male	212	37	17.5
Female	77	12	15.6
Age			
18-25	52	17	32.7**
26-34	74	9	12.2
35-45	110	17	15.5
46+	53	6	11.3
Education			
< 12	85	17	20.0
12	121	23	19.0
> 12	81	9	11.1
Marital Status			
Married	73	10	13.7
Never married	116	28	24.1*
Other	99	11	11.0
Employed			
No	76	17	22.4
Yes	212	32	15.1
Family Fighting			
Frequent (1-2 times/week)	53	17	32.1**
Sometimes (1-3 times/month)	75	17	22.7
Did not fight in the past month	145	13	9.0
Social Support			
No	52	14	26.9**
Yes	236	14	14.4
Church Attendance			
Never/Once	142	31	21.8*
Often	145	18	12.4
Neighborhood Safety			
Very safe	155	24	15.5
Somewhat safe	109	21	19.3
Not safe at all	21	4	19.0

Note: Sample sizes in some categories may not add to 289 due to missing data. Percents represent the proportion of individuals with a particular characteristic that used drugs out of the total number of individuals with the corresponding characteristic. For example, the 37 males that used drugs correspond to 17.5% of all the males in the study (37/212) and the 12 females correspond to 15.6% of all the females in the study (12/77). $* p < 0.05$ $** p < 0.01$.

TABLE 2. Association Between Family Fighting and Drug Use: Results of Multiple Logistic Regression

Characteristic	Drug Use	
	OR	95% CI
Age		
18-25	Reference	--
26-34	0.39	0.14-1.09
35-45	0.54	0.21-1.40
46+	0.68	0.20-2.34
Marital Status		
Married	Reference	
Never married	1.67	0.67-4.11
Other	0.84	0.31-2.23
Family Fighting		
No fights	Reference	
Sometimes	2.80	1.21-6.45
Frequent	4.53	1.89-10.82
Social Support		
No	Reference	
Yes	0.49	1.00-1.13
Church Attendance		
Never/Once	Reference	
Often	0.60	0.29-1.21

information is missing on the interaction between the type of drug used and family violence.

Nonetheless, these findings highlight the important association that exists between a recovering person's relationship with his or her family and sobriety. The findings also highlight the role that social support, including church attendance may play in a person's recovery. Given these findings an integrated model of practice may be required to address the significance of these issues as they impact many of the same families. Each practice area, substance abuse, domestic violence and child welfare, possesses distinctive boundaries and patterns. However, interaction between the systems must occur and targeted interventions must be multi-disciplinary.

The availability of social support was found to be inversely associated with drug use. As such, it is important for practitioners to be aware of the importance of support system utilization in the general population and in particular among individuals of various cultures. Reliance on extended family members as a means of social support is a more salient structure for African-Americans than for Caucasians (Hunter, 1997). Scannapieco and Jackson (1996) found that within the African-American community increased kinship care was a resilient response to stressors experienced by the family. The authors define resilience as "the overcoming of some risk factor resulting in positive adaptation" (p. 191). This resilience is seen as a way in which to preserve the extended family. Considerable heterogeneity exists across Latino populations on family functioning due to variation on social class, immigration status, geographic residence, and acculturation, among others (Zuniga, 1992). Nonetheless, the value of family interdependence found among Latino populations could either benefit the individual as a result of the extended support system or be a detriment to the recovery process by not allowing the individual to change.

Research also has shown that individuals from other minority populations also turn frequently to this natural helping system to fulfill their emotional and tangible needs (Leslie, 1992; Hanline & Daley, 1992; Koyano, Hashimoto, Fukawa, Shibata & Gunji, 1994). The extent that family functioning and interpersonal processes facilitate or hinder recovery has not been investigated thoroughly among racial/ethnic minority families. A recent study of the effects of family involvement on an individual's recovery among Native Hawaiian and other Pacific and Asian women provide some evidence of the importance of including a member of the extended family in the recovery process (Morelli & Fong, 2000).

Easton et al. (2000) assert that "When assessing the relationship between substance abuse and family violence, it is important to target both issues in an integrated way" (p. 24). To help alleviate these issues, as supported by this study's findings, the authors suggest the following practice changes:

- Comprehensive training for front-line staff within each practice area about the inter-relatedness of these issues;
- Coordinate simultaneous treatment plans for families experiencing multiple problems;
- Enhance family therapy programs to address these issues within the family structure;
- Conducting follow-up sessions and/or aftercare with families to ensure treatment successes are maintained.

Research

Further research into the overlap of family fighting and drug use may include the following:

- As with many illnesses, the pattern of drug abuse may have points of remission (i.e., sobriety) and relapse along a continuum. Therefore, the cross-sectional nature of this study's design does not allow us to determine the temporal association between this cycle and family fighting. Thus, it is recommended that a longitudinal design be employed to determine the variables which may trigger a relapse and/or fight.
- It is hypothesized that some drugs may contribute differentially to one's level of violence. Therefore, more detailed research into the specific drugs utilized, as well as their interaction effect, and its impact on family fighting will be beneficial in identifying more targeted treatments. Controlling for co-occurring disorders must also be considered. Simultaneously, the mechanisms by which family interaction influences a person's likelihood of resuming drug use needs to be further investigated.
- In general, social supports may be conceptualized as a 2 by 3 matrix consisting of two sources and three functions of social support (Vaux, 1988; Zarit, Pearlin & Schaie, 1993). Sources of social support may consist of informal and/or formal sources (Zarit et al., 1993); with three categories (emotional, informational and tangible support) most consistently highlighted (see Gottlieb, 1981 or Lin, 1986 for a typological review). In assisting clients to maintain sobriety, as well as reducing the occurrence of family fighting, it is important to examine these various social support factors to determine which permutations may be the most beneficial along the family life cycle.

CONCLUSION

Society has a vested interest in the welfare of its families. Family fighting and substance abuse have numerous linkages to other problems for society, such as increased health care and other costs, increased juvenile delinquency and poor school performance. In addition, the children of these families are reported to be at increased risk for an array of behavioral, emotional and cognitive problems, as well as abusing substances themselves (Sheridan, 1995). Preventing further drug use not only benefits the individual but may also help prevent the intergenerational transmission of this maladaptive behavior.

REFERENCES

Benshoff, J.J., & Janikowski, T.P. (2000). The rehabilitation model of substance abuse counseling. Belmont, CA: Brooks Cole.

Besinger, B., Garland, A., Litrownik, A., & Landsverk, J. (1999). Caregiver substance abuse among maltreated children placed in out-of-home care. *Child Welfare, LXXVIII*(2), 221-239.

Black, R., & Mayer, J. (1980). Parents with special problems: Alcoholism and opiate addiction. *Child Abuse and Neglect, 4,* 45-54.

Bureau of Justice Statistics. (1994). *Fact sheet: Drug-related crime.* Rockville, MD: Drugs and Crime Data Center and Clearinghouse.

Corvo, K., & Carpenter, E. (2000). Effects of parental substance abuse on current levels of domestic violence: A possible elaboration of intergenerational transmission processes. *Journal of Family Violence, 15*(2), 123-135.

Delva, J., Allgood, J., Morrell, R., & McNeece, C. A. (in press). A state-wide follow-up study of alcohol and illegal drug use treatment. *Research on Social Work Practice.*

Easton, C., Swan, S., & Sinha, R. (2000). Prevalence of family violence in clients entering substance abuse treatment. *Journal of Substance Abuse Treatment, 18,* 23-28.

Friedman, A. (1998). Substance use/abuse as a predictor to illegal and violent behavior: A review of the relevant literature. *Aggression and Violent Behavior, 3*(4), 339-355.

Gorney, B. (1989). Domestic violence and chemical dependency: Dual problems, dual interventions. *Journal of Psychoactive Drugs, 21,* 229-238.

Gottlieb, B. (1981). *Social networks and social supports.* Beverly Hills, CA: Sage.

Hanline, M., & Daley, S. (1992). Family coping strategies and strengths in Hispanic, African-American, and Caucasian families of young children. *Topics in Early Childhood Special Education, 12,* 351-366.

Holtzworth-Munroe, A., & Stuart, G. (1994). Typologies of male batterers: Three subtypes and the differences among them. *Psychological Bulletin, 116,* 476-497.

Hubbard, R. L., Marsden, M. E., Rachal, J. V., Harwood, H. J., Cavanaugh, E. R., & Ginzburg, H. M. (1989). *Drug abuse treatment: A national study on effectiveness.* Chapel Hill, NC: University of North Carolina Press.

Hunter, A. G. (1997). Counting on grandmothers: Black mothers' and fathers' reliance on grandmothers for parenting support. *Journal of Family Issues, 18*(3), 251-269.

Koyano, W., Hashimoto, M., Fukawa, T., Shibata, H., & Gunji, A. (1994). The social support system of Japanese elderly. *Journal of Cross-Cultural Gerontology, 9,* 323-333.

Leslie, L. (1992). The role of informal support networks in the adjustment of Central American immigrant families. *Journal of Community Psychology, 20,* 243-256.

Lin, N. (1986). Conceptualizing social support. In N. Lin, A. Dean & W. Ensel (Eds.), *Social Support, Life Events, and Depression* (pp. 17-30). New York: Academic Press.

Maiden, R. (1997). Alcohol dependence and domestic violence: Incidence and treatment implications. *Alcoholism Treatment Quarterly, 15* (2), 31-50.

Morelli, P.T., & Fong, R. (2000). The role of Hawaiian elders in substance abuse treatment among Asian/Pacific Islander women. In J. Delva (Ed.), *Substance abuse issues among families in diverse populations* (pp. 33-44). New York: The Haworth Press, Inc.

Scannapieco, M., & Jackson, S. (1996). Kinship care: The African-American response to family preservation. *Social Work, 41*(2), 190-195.

Sheridan, M. (1995). A proposed intergenerational model of substance abuse, family functioning, and abuse/neglect. *Child Abuse and Neglect, 19*(5), 519-530.

Stanton, M.D. (1978). The family and drug misuse: A bibliography. *American Journal of Drug and Alcohol Abuse, 5,* 151-170.

Stanton, M.D. (1980). Some overlooked aspects of the family and drug abuse. In B.G. Ellis (Ed.), *Drug abuse from the family perspective* (ADM 80-910). Washington, DC.: National Institute on Drug Abuse.

Substance Abuse and Mental Health Services Administration. (1998). *Services research outcome study.* DHHS Publication No. (SMA) 98-3177. Rockville, MD: Author.

Vaux, A. (1988). *Social support: Theory, research, and intervention.* New York: Praeger.

Wolock, I., & Magura, S. (1996). Parental substance abuse as a predictor of child maltreatment re-reports *Child Abuse and Neglect, 20*(12), 1183-1193.

Zarit, S., Pearlin, L., & Schaie, K. (1993). *Caregiving systems: Informal and formal helpers.* Hillsdale, NJ: L. Erlbaum Associates.

Zuniga, M. (1992). Families with Latino roots. In E.W. Lynch & M.J. Hanson (Eds.), Developing cross-cultural competence (pp. 151-179). Baltimore, MD: Paul H. Brookes Publishing, Co.

Parental Involvement, Needs and Drug-Related Service Utilization Among Mexican Middle and High School Students

Fernando A. Wagner, ScD
Guilherme Borges, ScD
María Elena Medina-Mora, PhD
Corina Benjet, PhD
Jorge A. Villatoro, MSc

SUMMARY. *Introduction:* Very little research has been done in Mexico to estimate drug-related treatment needs or service utilization. There

Fernando A. Wagner, Guilherme Borges, María Elena Medina-Mora, Corina Benjet, and Jorge A. Villatoro are affiliated with Instituto Nacional de Psiquiatría, Dirección de Investigaciones Epidemiológicas y Psicosociales, Mexico.

Address correspondence to: Dr. Fernando A. Wagner, Instituto Nacional de Psiquiatría, Dirección de Investigaciones Epidemiológicas y Psicosociales. Calz. México Xochimilco # 101, Colonia San Lorenzo Huipulco, Delegación Tlalpan, C.P. 14370, México, D.F. Mexico (E-mail: fernanw@imp.edu.mx).

The authors of this paper wish to gratefully acknowledge Héctor Cardiel and Clara Fleiz, who played an important role in the development of the 1997 survey of drug use among middle and high school students of the Federal District in Mexico.

During the preparation of this paper, Dr. Wagner received support from the National Council on Science and Technology of Mexico (CONACYT), Repatriation grant # 000358. The 1997 survey of drug use among middle and high school students of the Federal District in Mexico was funded with grants 3431P-H from CONACYT and 4320/97 from the Instituto Nacional de Psiquiatría.

[Haworth co-indexing entry note]: "Parental Involvement, Needs and Drug-Related Service Utilization Among Mexican Middle and High School Students." Wagner et al. Co-published simultaneously in *Journal of Family Social Work* (The Haworth Social Work Practice Press, an imprint of The Haworth Press. Inc.) Vol. 6, No. 1, 2001, pp. 79-95; and: *Families and Health: Cross-Cultural Perspectives* (ed: Jorge Delva) The Haworth Social Work Practice Press, an imprint of The Haworth Press, Inc., 2001, pp. 79-95. Single or multiple copies of this article are available for a fee from The Haworth Document Delivery Service [1-800-342-9678, 9:00 a.m. - 5:00 p.m. (EST). E-mail address: getinfo@haworthpressinc.com].

is also scarce epidemiological research on the influence of parents on drug-related service utilization by adolescents in Mexico. In this paper, we use advanced epidemiologic strategies to provide population-based estimates of the association between parental involvement and treatment needs and service utilization, by level of drug use, with and without adjustment for sociodemographic characteristics. *Methods:* We used data from the latest survey on drug use, representative of all middle and high school students in the Federal District of Mexico (Mexico City). A standardized, self-administered questionnaire was given to 10,173 students aged 12-22 (mean = 14.6, SE = 0.08), especially designed to assess use of several drugs and risk/protective factors, including a sub-scale on parental involvement. All analyses used procedures that account for the complex sample design. *Results:* Students with lower parental involvement (lowest quartile) were found to be more likely to have used drugs in their lifetime, in the past year, as well as in the past month. Moreover, students with the lowest quartile of parental involvement were more likely to have used two or more drugs in their lifetime, and this association was estimated to be independent of sex, age, school enrollment in the past year as well as history of working part or full time in the prior year. About 20% of the students who ever used two or more drugs received some drug-related help, however 50-55% reported they would like to use drugs less. Service utilization was associated with higher numbers of drugs ever used, but not with higher levels of parental involvement. *Discussion:* Parental involvement seems to play a major role as a protective factor against drug use initiation among students, but does not differentiate drug users who seek help from those who do not. Further research is needed to answer whether this is due to students with higher levels of parental involvement having less problematic patterns of drug use. The discrepancy between wanting to use drugs less and service utilization points to the need for further research into the factors that may influence service utilization and, ultimately, recovery. *[Article copies available for a fee from The Haworth Document Delivery Service: 1-800-342-9678. E-mail address: <getinfo@haworthpressinc.com> Website: <http://www.HaworthPress.com> © 2001 by The Haworth Press, Inc. All rights reserved.]*

KEYWORDS. Treatment, adolescents, substance use, needs assessment, epidemiology

INTRODUCTION

For many years, the scope of drug use and drug use problems among Mexican students was stable. However, new patterns have emerged recently that warrant proper public health interventions. These changes include an increase in the proportion of students who have used two or more drugs, an increase in the number and proportion of students who have tried cocaine, and an increase in the proportion of young females who have become users of cocaine (Rojas et al., 1998; Villatoro et al., 1999). Surveillance systems have detected an excess of cocaine use and cocaine-related mentions in treatment centers, and young offenders (Ortiz et al., 1999). However, very little research has been done in Mexico to estimate drug-related treatment needs and service utilization among the general population. Sooner or later, these changes in drug use in Mexico will affect the demand for treatment. Thus, it is imperative to have representative estimates of the proportion of substance users who use health services among the general population. According to prior research, it is expected that this proportion will be low (Goldberg & Huxley, 1992; Solís & Medina-Mora, 1994; Marino et al, 1995; Katz et al., 1997), and that there is a considerable time-lag between onset of the problem and treatment-seeking (Gater et al., 1991; Lara & Acevedo, 1996).

Because adolescent students are still dependents of their parents, an important issue in adolescent service utilization, not just in Mexico, but in the international literature, relates to the influence of parental involvement and adolescent-parent relations on service utilization for drug problems. Several studies with adolescents and school aged children in the United States and Sweden lend evidence to support a relationship between parenting variables (such as monitoring, involvement, communication, affect) and adolescent problem behavior in general (e.g., Richardson et al., 1993; Nelson, Patience, & MacDonald, 1999) and drug use in particular (e.g., Chilcoat, Dishion & Anthony, 1995, Dishion & Loeber, 1985; Stronski et al., 2000). Yet, we do not know how parents influence their adolescents' utilization of drug-related services.

Therefore, in this paper, we use advanced epidemiologic strategies to provide population-based estimates of the proportion of students who have used drug-related services, and of the association between parental involvement, treatment needs and service utilization, by level of drug use.

METHODS

We used data from the latest survey of drug use, representative of all middle school students in the Federal District of Mexico (a.k.a. Mexico

City). Detailed descriptions of this and prior surveys have been published elsewhere (among other papers, see Medina-Mora et al., 1993; Rojas et al., 1998; Villatoro et al., 1999). Briefly, the survey belongs to a systematic effort on surveillance of drug use among Mexican students conducted by the Ministry of Education and the National Institute of Psychiatry over the past 20 years. For the 1997 survey, the sample frame comprised all students who were enrolled in middle and high school at the beginning of the 1997-98 academic year (grades 7 through 12 in the U.S.), which number close to 1.5 million students (Banamex, 1998).

The sample was designed to provide estimates of drug use representative of each of the 16 districts that comprise the Federal District. The sample was selected using a multi-stage procedure, the first stage consisting of the selection of schools within districts, and the second stage being the selection of groups within schools. Out of the 12,170 students who were expected to participate, a total of 10,173 students actually took part in the survey, resulting in an 83.6% of the total number of students expected to be surveyed. In the sample, 51.9% of the students were females and 48.1% were males. Most students were 14 years or younger (54%), with a mean age of 14.6 (SE = 0.08), and were enrolled in middle school (61%), or high school (27.6%) at the time of assessment. However, because of this paper's focus on parental involvement, we restricted the analytical sample to students younger than 21 years who had provided data on key variables. This restriction resulted in a final analytical sample of 9,466 respondents, after exclusion of 163 students who were older than 20 (1.6%) and 544 students who had missing data in key variables (5.4%).

A standardized, self-administered questionnaire was used for the 1997 survey, similar to the core instrument that has been used in prior surveys (Medina-Mora et al., 1981). The questionnaire gathers data about use of alcohol, tobacco, amphetamines, tranquilizers, marihuana, cocaine, crack-cocaine, inhalants, hallucinogens, sedatives, and heroin. For each of these drugs, data were obtained for lifetime, past year, and past month usage, as well as the number of times each of these drugs were used in their lifetime. As an indicator of drug involvement, we constructed a variable counting the number of drugs that had ever been used by each student. Service needs and utilization was measured by asking the following questions: "Have you seen a physician or talked to a school counselor, or have you been in a hospital due to drug use, excluding alcohol and tobacco?" as well as "Do your parents think that you use drugs too frequently (not including alcohol and tobacco)?" and

"Would you like to use less drugs than you currently do (not including alcohol and tobacco)?" Possible answers to these questions are: yes/no/I don't use drugs.

As a part of data on several risk/protective factors, a set of items with four Likert-like scale options was included regarding family relations, communication and environment, which had been previously designed and tested (Villatoro et al., 1997). We selected seven items on communication with parents as well as parental support and encouragement to test the hypothesis that higher parental involvement would be associated with increased service utilization among students who had used drugs. These items are listed below:

Items included in the sub-scale of parental involvement:

1. When something personal worries me, I talk with my parents about it
2. I talk with my parents regarding things that happened during the day
3. I like talking with my parents about my personal problems
4. My parents motivate me to keep going when I am troubled
5. My parents are supportive when I start something new
6. I talk with my parents about my personal problems
7. My parents make me feel comfortable talking about my personal problems

The scale's reliability was found to be very good (alpha = 0.86), and exploratory factor analysis yielded a one-factor solution with an Eigenvalue of 3.27 and all item loadings close to or above 0.60. Based on this information, we created a score by adding the answers to each of the seven questions. Because we expected to observe a curvilinear relation between parental involvement and service utilization, we decided to create variables indicating quartiles of parental involvement, and use the lowest quartile of parental involvement as a comparison or reference group.

Data analysis was performed as follows. First, we prepared a cross-tabulation of students by number of drugs used in their lifetime, past year, and past month, according to parental involvement and socioeconomic characteristics. Then, we estimated the association between number of drugs used and parental involvement, with and without statistical adjustment for potential imbalances in socioeconomic characteristics. Number of drugs used was recoded into ordinal categories as "never used drugs," "used one drug," and "used two or more drugs." Attending to the ordinal nature of the outcome, a polytomous (ordinal) logistic regression model was implemented. Then, selecting students who had used one or more drugs, we estimated service needs and utilization by number of drugs used and tested the association of service needs and utilization with parental involvement and number of drugs used, with and without statistical adjustment of socioeconomic characteristics. Again, selecting only those students who reported having used two or more drugs, we have prepared a cross-tabulation to illustrate similarities and differences between groups of students defined by whether they used drug-related services or not, by parental involvement and socioeconomic characteristics. All analyses took into consideration the complex sample design of the study using STATA software (Stata Corp., 1999).

RESULTS

An estimated 6.3% of students were estimated to have used one drug in their lifetime, 4.7% used two or more drugs, and 88.0% had never used drugs. As shown in Table 1, students with higher levels of parental involvement (i.e., fourth quartile) used fewer drugs in their lifetime, last year, and past month, compared to students with lower levels of parental involvement (first quartile). Table 1 also shows that a higher proportion of males than females have used drugs, and the difference is larger for the use of two or more drugs during one's lifetime, past year, and past month. As expected, proportions of drug use are higher for older students, and the age difference somewhat diminishes as the window of observation is smaller and closer to assessment (e.g., lifetime, last year, and past month).

Table 2 presents estimates of the association between number of drugs used and parental involvement, accounting simultaneously for sex, age, past year school enrollment, and past year work enrollment. Compared to the lowest quartile, students with higher levels of parental involvement were estimated to be half as likely to have used one drug (adjusted Odds Ratio, $OR = 0.65$, 0.47, and 0.39, for the second, third, and fourth quartile, respectively, with 95% Confidence Intervals (95% CI) that ranged from 0.32 to 0.77). In turn, students with higher levels of parental involvement were estimated to be half as likely to have used two or more drugs, compared to students in the lowest quartile of parental involvement who have never used drugs or have used only one drug

TABLE 1. Parental involvement and sociodemographic characteristics of students, by number of drugs used in their lifetime, last year, and past month (n = 9,466)

| | Lifetime | | | | | | Drugs Used Last Year | | | | | | Past Month | | | | | | Total | |
| | Never | | One | | Two or more | | None | | One | | Two or more | | None | | One | | Two or more | | | |
	#	%	#	%	#	%	#	%	#	%	#	%	#	%	#	%	#	%	#	%
Quartile of Parental Involvement																				
First (lowest)	1972	83.31	212	8.96	183	7.73	2097	88.59	164	6.93	106	4.48	2209	93.32	117	4.94	41	1.73	2367	100.00
Second	2098	88.67	150	6.34	118	4.99	2177	92.01	126	5.33	63	2.66	2281	96.41	61	2.58	24	1.01	2366	100.00
Third	2151	90.91	130	5.49	85	3.59	2224	94.00	97	4.10	45	1.90	2307	97.51	43	1.82	16	0.68	2366	100.00
Fourth	2201	92.99	108	4.56	58	2.45	2264	95.65	73	3.08	30	1.27	2323	98.14	36	1.52	8	0.34	2367	100.00
Sex																				
Male	3851	86.25	320	7.17	294	6.58	4061	90.95	244	5.46	160	3.58	4259	95.39	144	3.23	62	1.39	4465	100.00
Female	4571	91.40	280	5.60	150	3.00	4701	94.00	216	4.32	84	1.68	4861	97.20	113	2.26	27	0.54	5001	100.00
Age																				
12 or less	1429	95.27	49	3.27	22	1.47	1458	97.20	30	2.00	12	0.80	1481	98.73	14	0.93	5	0.33	1500	100.00
13	1620	93.05	79	4.54	42	2.41	1662	95.46	57	3.27	22	1.26	1699	97.59	36	2.07	6	0.34	1741	100.00
14	1713	89.92	120	6.30	72	3.78	1763	92.55	88	4.62	54	2.83	1832	96.17	52	2.73	21	1.10	1905	100.00
15	1367	87.46	107	6.85	89	5.69	1424	91.11	90	5.76	49	3.13	1492	95.46	52	3.33	19	1.22	1563	100.00
16	1020	86.44	91	7.71	69	5.85	1074	91.02	72	6.10	34	2.88	1126	95.42	42	3.56	17	1.02	1180	100.00
17	749	83.69	85	9.50	61	6.82	799	89.27	60	6.70	36	4.02	852	95.20	26	2.91	17	1.90	895	100.00
18	335	79.38	40	9.48	47	11.14	360	85.31	44	10.43	18	4.27	391	92.65	28	6.64	3	0.71	422	100.00
19 or more	189	72.69	29	11.15	42	16.15	222	85.38	19	7.31	19	7.31	247	95.00	7	2.69	6	2.31	260	100.00
Past year school status																				
Did not study	447	81.72	42	7.678	58	10.60	472	86.29	44	8.04	31	5.67	500	91.41	34	6.22	13	2.38	547	100.00
Part time	1010	84.52	98	8.20	87	7.28	1060	88.70	85	7.11	50	4.18	1133	94.81	46	3.85	16	1.34	1195	100.00
Full time	6961	90.17	460	5.959	299	3.87	7226	93.60	331	4.29	163	2.11	7483	96.93	177	2.29	60	0.78	7720	100.00
Past year work status																				
Did not work	7341	90.46	474	5.841	300	3.70	7596	93.60	355	4.37	164	2.02	7869	96.97	191	2.35	55	0.68	8115	100.00
Part time	627	79.57	71	9.01	90	11.42	675	85.66	57	7.23	56	7.11	728	92.39	37	4.70	23	2.92	788	100.00
Full time	336	79.62	40	9.479	46	10.90	361	85.55	40	9.48	21	4.98	386	91.47	26	6.16	10	2.37	422	100.00

TABLE 2. Estimated association between number of drugs used (none, one, two or more), parental involvement, and sociodemographic covariates. Results from ordered logistic regression analyses (n = 9,321)

Characteristic	Lifetime		Past Year		Last Month	
	OR	95% CI	OR	95% CI	OR	95% CI
Quartile of Parental Involvement						
Second	0.65	0.54-0.77	0.69	0.56-0.84	0.56	0.42-0.74
Third	0.47	0.39-0.57	0.48	0.38-0.59	0.33	0.24-0.47
Fourth	0.39	0.32-0.48	0.37	0.29-0.48	0.30	0.21-0.43
First (lowest)	1.00	---	1.00	---	1.00	---
Sex						
Male	1.53	1.32-1.78	1.39	1.17-1.65	1.47	1.17-1.86
Female	1.00	---	1.00	---	1.00	---
Age	1.26	1.21-1.31	1.22	1.17-1.27	1.15	1.09-1.22
Past year school status						
Part time	1.21	0.99-1.47	1.37	1.10-1.71	1.25	0.91-1.72
Did not study	1.27	0.98-1.65	1.46	1.10-1.93	1.89	1.33-2.70
Full time	1.00	---	1.00	---	1.00	---
Past year work status						
Part time	1.61	1.32-1.95	1.66	1.31-2.09	1.81	1.31-2.49
Full time	1.46	1.10-1.95	1.42	1.03-1.96	1.62	1.09-2.41
Did not work	1.00	---	1.00	---	1.00	---

in their lifetime, past year, and past month (the *OR* and 95% CI are the same, as one coefficient summarizes the association). This inverse association between drug use and quartile of parental involvement was found to be statistically significant for drug use in one's lifetime, past year, as well as past month. In addition, higher levels of parental involvement were estimated to be associated with lower number of drugs used, among students who had used at least one drug (p = 0.0423). More specifically, among students who had used drugs in their lifetime, those with the highest quartile of parental involvement were estimated to be 30% less likely to have used two or more drugs than students in the lowest quartile (p = 0.019). A similar finding was obtained for students in the second highest quartile of parental involvement, though the evidence is marginally significant in statistical terms (p = 0.056).

Approximately, eight to eleven percent of students who used one drug reported to have used drug-related services, and 19% to 23% of students who used two or more drugs did so, as shown in Table 3. Only one in five students who used two or more drugs in the past month reported that his/her parents believe she or he uses drugs too much. However, an overwhelming 50% of students who have used two or more drugs in their lifetime reported they would like to use drugs less, and the percentage was higher for students who used drugs in the past year and in the past month (53% and 55% respectively). In this context, it is interesting to note that only 22% of the students who had used two or more drugs in the past month reported their parents believe they use drugs too much (Table 3).

Table 4 shows estimates of the association between lifetime drug-related service needs and utilization and several covariates among students who had used drugs (students who have not used drugs are not included). In general, the analysis fails to show a statistically significant association between parental involvement and service needs and utilization. However, a few differences were observed that are noteworthy. Compared to the lowest quartile, students with the second quartile of parental involvement were estimated to be 1.7 times more likely to have

TABLE 3. Indicators of drug services needs and utilization among students who used drugs, by number of drugs used at different time periods

Number of drugs used	Received drug related services					Parents believe too much drug use					Would like to use drugs less				
	No		Yes		Total	No		Yes		Total	No		Yes		Total
	#	%	#	%	#	#	%	#	%	#	#	%	#	%	#
Lifetime															
One drug	537	92.11	46	7.89	583	314	97.52	8	2.48	322	114	87.69	16	12.31	130
Two or more	351	81.25	81	18.75	432	317	89.30	38	10.70	355	99	50.00	99	50.00	198
Last year															
One drug	401	89.71	46	10.29	447	426	96.60	15	3.40	441	144	79.12	38	20.88	182
Two or more	189	79.75	48	20.25	237	205	86.86	31	13.14	236	69	47.26	77	52.74	146
Past month															
One drug	221	88.76	28	11.24	249	234	93.98	15	6.02	249	174	72.20	67	27.80	241
Two or more	68	77.27	20	22.73	88	68	78.16	19	21.84	87	39	44.83	48	55.17	87

TABLE 4. Estimated association between drug services needs and utilization, parental involvement, number of used drugs, and sociodemographic covariates, among students who used drugs

Characteristic	Received drug related services		Parents believe too much drug use		Would like to use drugs less	
				Yes		
	OR	95% CI	OR	95% CI	OR	95% CI
Quartile of Parental Involvement						
Second	1.73	1.08-2.77	0.77	0.40-1.49	0.66	0.43-1.02
Third	1.02	0.58-1.80	0.57	0.25-1.28	0.98	0.64-1.48
Fourth	1.04	0.57-1.90	0.74	0.32-1.73	0.49	0.29-0.84
First (lowest)	1.00	---	1.00	---	1.00	---
Lifetime drugs used						
Two or more	2.73	1.84-4.07	3.53	1.93-6.47	7.64	5.32-10.97
One drug	1.00	---	1.00	---	1.00	---
Sex						
Male	1.03	0.68-1.58	1.31	0.71-2.42	2.24	1.53-3.28
Female	1.00	---	1.00	---	1.00	---
Age						
Each year compared to the prior year	0.98	0.88-1.09	1.02	0.88-1.18	0.99	0.91-1.08
Past year school status						
Part time	1.00	0.59-1.72	1.04	0.50-2.15	0.86	0.56-1.32
Did not study	0.82	0.39-1.71	1.24	0.49-3.16	0.98	0.56-1.73
Full time	1.00	---	1.00	---	1.00	---
Past year work status						
Part time	1.93	1.15-3.24	0.85	0.38-1.90	1.13	0.73-1.76
Full time	1.69	0.80-3.55	1.34	0.47-3.80	0.65	0.33-1.29
Did not work	1.00	---	1.00	---	1.00	---

received drug-related services (OR = 1.73, 95% CI, 1.08-2.77). As predicted, the strongest association of drug-related service utilization was found with having used two or more drugs, as compared to students who used only one drug in their lifetime (OR = 2.73, 95 CI, 1.84-4.07), and this association was even stronger with regard to parental belief that their child was using drugs too much (OR = 3.53, 95 CI, 1.93-6.47), as well as with the desire of using drugs less (OR = 7.64, 95 CI, 5.32-10.97). An interesting observation is that sex was not estimated to be associated with service utilization or parental belief of too much drug use.

Although we anticipated the possibility of sub-group variation in the association of parental involvement with drug-related service utilization by sex, in general, the analyses did not substantiate this possibility (p > 0.05). However, some male-female differences were found with regard to the desire to use drugs less. Males were estimated to be twice as likely to endorse they would like to use drugs less (*OR* = 2.24, 95% CI, 1.53-3.28), and a significant interaction was found involving the desire to use drugs less, sex, and parental involvement. Specifically, female students who had used drugs and had higher levels of parental involvement were less likely to report they would like to use drugs less, especially compared to the corresponding estimates for males (p < 0.05).

Table 5 describes characteristics of students who used two or more drugs in their lifetime, by whether or not they have received drug-related services. The number of respondents becomes too small when several attributes are analyzed simultaneously, even with samples as large as the one we use for this study, which has prevented us from applying more advanced statistical tools. Descriptive analyses of characteristics of students who used services and those who did not failed to show differences at conventional levels of statistical significance (p < 0.05).

DISCUSSION

The most important findings of this study can be summarized as follows: (1) students with lower parental involvement (lowest quartile) were found to be more likely to have used drugs in their lifetime, in the past year, as well as in the past month. Moreover, students with the lowest quartile of parental involvement were more likely to have used two or more drugs in their lifetime, and this association was estimated to be independent of sex, age, school enrollment in the past year as well as history of working part or full time in the prior year; (2) about 19% of the students who ever used two or more drugs received some drug-related help, however 50-55% reported they would like to use drugs less; and (3) service utilization among students who had used drugs was associated with having used two or more drugs in the lifetime, but not with higher levels of parental involvement.

Before discussing these findings in detail, it is important to acknowledge several limitations of this study. First, the cross-sectional nature of the data makes it difficult to sort the sequence of events without ambiguity. For example, drug use initiation or escalation could lead to more

TABLE 5. Characteristics of students who used two or more drugs in their lifetime, by drug-related services utilization

| | Received services | | | | | |
| | No | | Yes | | Total | |
	#	%	#	%	#	%
Quartile of Parental Involvement						
First (lowest)	145	84.80	26	15.20	171	100.00
Second	89	76.07	28	23.93	117	100.00
Third	67	81.71	15	18.29	82	100.00
Fourth	42	77.78	12	22.22	54	100.00
Sex						
Male	116	84.06	22	15.94	138	100.00
Female	227	79.37	59	20.63	286	100.00
Age						
12 or less	17	80.95	4	19.05	21	100.00
13	32	80.00	8	20.00	40	100.00
14	52	75.36	17	24.64	69	100.00
15	65	81.25	15	18.75	80	100.00
16	56	83.58	11	16.42	67	100.00
17	50	83.33	10	16.67	60	100.00
18	37	82.22	8	17.78	45	100.00
19 or more	34	80.95	8	19.05	42	100.00
Past year school status						
Did not study	228	81.14	53	18.86	281	100.00
Part time	69	81.18	16	18.82	85	100.00
Full time	46	79.31	12	20.69	58	100.00
Past year work status						
Did not work	243	83.51	48	16.49	291	100.00
Part time	64	73.56	23	26.44	87	100.00
Full time	36	78.26	10	21.74	46	100.00

intensive parent monitoring or to an emergence of family conflicts, but also it is possible that higher parental involvement might have served as a buffering factor against risky situations that might otherwise have ended in initiation or greater drug involvement. Longitudinal data is needed here to clarify the direction of the association. Also, it is important to acknowledge that self-report data is subject to assumptions on completeness and accuracy. This survey did not include other measurement methods, however, it is important to mention several steps that were taken in order to promote good quality in the data. These steps included intensive and systematic training of staff administering the survey to students, reassurance of the confidentiality of the data, and inclusion of detailed instructions for each section of the survey.

Finally, it is important to note that findings from this study may or may not apply to youth who are not enrolled in middle or high school. Further research is certainly needed for those not enrolled in school, especially considering empirical evidence of excess risk for drug use among school dropouts in Mexico (Rosovsky et al., 1999; Medina-Mora et al., 1999).

Notwithstanding these and other limitations, the present study provides novel information that may be useful in the context of research on needs assessment and service utilization. We found parental involvement to be negatively associated with lower odds of using drugs. This is consistent with a body of evidence linking parental involvement with reduced likelihood of several negative outcomes, such as drug use (Dishion & Loeber, 1985; Richardson et al., 1993; Chilcoat et al., 1995; Chilcoat & Anthony, 1996) and points to parent education as an important avenue for intervention to prevent drug use initiation among children. On the other hand, we did not find differences of parental involvement by number of drugs used (i.e., one versus two or more drugs). Other researchers however have found peers to be especially important for initiation into marijuana use, while parental factors gained in importance in the transition from marijuana use to the use of other illicit drugs (Kandel, 1985; Hoffman, 1993; Stronski et al., 2000). Methodological and cultural differences need to be taken into consideration in order to explain these differing findings. One possibility is the different parental factors employed. Some measures reflect more parental monitoring while others reflect parental communication and affective tone of the parent-adolescent relationship. Also, it is possible that risk/protective factors vary across stages of drug involvement, as discussed by Glanz and Pickens (1992), and more specifically by Clayton (1992). Parental involvement among Mexican students might be associated with reduced likelihood of initiating drug use, but other factors such as peer drug use and deviant peer association might play a more important role with regard to escalation of drug use.

The finding that only 22% of parents with children who have used two or more drugs in the past month reported to view this drug usage as too much, leads one to wonder how much parents are aware of their children's drug use and how much knowledge they have of the problems associated with drug use. Further research is needed to understand the extent of the disconnect that exists between what parents think their children are doing and the children's actual drug use.

While we found service utilization to be associated with higher number of drugs ever used, we failed to find a significant association with parental involvement. Many studies have documented health services utilization to be associated with higher levels of psychiatric morbidity and comorbidity, though an important proportion of cases with mental disorders does not get services at all (e.g., Goldberg & Huxley, 1980, 1992; Offer et al., 1991; Marino et al., 1995; Katz et al., 1997; Medina-Mora et al., 1997). In this context, it is not surprising that students who have used two or more drugs were more likely to report having sought drug-related services than students who only used one drug. Also, it is important to consider that a study among Mexican-American students found that peers are the first source of help for drug-using children and adolescents, rather than their parents (Mason, 1997). Yet, it is also possible that adolescents with greater parental involvement develop less problematic patterns of drug use, which in turn is associated with reduced need of service utilization. A much larger sample and a prospective design would be needed to unravel these potential mechanisms.

The unfortunate discrepancy between desire to use less drugs and service utilization points to the importance of researching how best to reach adolescents in need, such as treatment availability, knowledge of treatment options, adolescent help-seeking strategies, and other mediating factors which might increase the likelihood of service utilization. The results of this article provide some empirical support which shed light on the last two questions. While number of drugs used increased the likelihood of receiving drug-related services, parental involvement, past school enrollment, and past year employment status did not.

Another important question is to whom drug-related services should be targeted. Based upon a foundation of epidemiological evidence on the person-to-person spread of drug initiation and the rapid transition from initial use to drug dependence, a recently published article makes the case for intervention at early stages of drug involvement, well before a more problematic pattern of drug use is developed (Anthony, 2000). Our research supports the idea that parent involvement (and thus targeting parents as well as adolescents in prevention/intervention programs) would be useful for Mexican youth during the early stages or before drug involvement. In Mexico, about one in five students in the Federal District who used two or more drugs have received some drug-related help. Yet, for each student who has received help there is another one who would like to use drugs less. If this is an indication of unmet treatment needs, further research is needed for a better understanding of factors that may influence service utilization and, ultimately, recovery. This might be helpful in reducing the spread of drug use, an urgent task in the face of the unfortunate changes in the epidemiology of drug use in Mexico.

REFERENCES

Anthony, J.C. (2000). Putting epidemiology and public health in needs assessment: drug dependence and beyond. In G. Andrews & S. Henderson (Eds.), *Unmet need in Psychiatry. Problems, resources, responses.* New York, NY: Cambridge University Press.

Banamex. *México Social 1996-1998. Estadísticas seleccionadas [Social Mexico 1996-1998. Selected statistics].* México D.F.: Banamex.

Chilcoat, H.D., Dishion, T.J., & Anthony J.C. (1995). Parent monitoring and the incidence of drug sampling in urban elementary school children. *American Journal of Epidemiology,* 141(1), 25-31.

Chilcoat, H.D., & Anthony, J.C. (1996). Impact of parent monitoring on initiation of drug use through late childhood. *Journal of the American Academy of Child & Adolescent Psychiatry,* 35(1), 91-100.

Clayton, R.R. (1992). Transitions in drug use: Risk and protective factors. In: M. Glanz & R.R. Pickens (Eds.), *Vulnerability to Drug Abuse.* Washington, D.C: American Psychological Association.

Dishion, T.J., & Loeber, R. (1985). Adolescent marijuana and alcohol use: The role of parents and peers revisited. *American Journal of Drug and Alcohol Abuse,* 11(1 & 2), 11-25.

Gater, R., Almeida e Sousa, D., Barrientos, G., Caraveo, J., Chandrashekar, C.R., Dhadphale, M., Goldberg, D., Al-Kathiri, A.H., Mubbashar, M., Silhan, K., Thong, D., Torres-Gonzalez, F., & Sartorious, N. (1991). The pathways to psychiatric care: A cross-cultural study. *Psychological Medicine,* 21: 761-774.

Glanz, M., & Pickens, R.R. (1992). *Vulnerability to Drug Abuse.* Washington, D.C.: American Psychological Association.

Goldberg, D., & Huxley, P. (1980). *Mental illness in the community: The pathway to psychiatric care.* London, U.K.: Tavistock Publications.

Goldberg, D., & Huxley, P. (1992). *Common Mental Disorders. A Bio-Social Model.* London: Tavistock/Routledge,

Hoffman, J.P. (1993). Exploring the direct and indirect family effects on adolescent drug use. *Journal of Drug Issues,* 23(3), 535-557.

Kandel, D.B. (1985). On processes of peer influences in adolescent drug use: a developmental perspective. *Advances in Alcohol & Substance Abuse,* 4(3-4), 139-163.

Katz, S.J., Kessler, R.C., Frank, R.G., Leaf, P., Lin, E., & Edlund, M. (1997). The use of outpatient mental health services in the United States and Ontario: The impact of mental morbidity and perceived need for care. *American Journal of Public Health*, 87(7), 1136-1143.

Lara, M.A., & Acevedo, M. (1996). Patrones de utilización de los servicios de salud mental [Patterns of mental health service utilization]. *Salud Mental*, 19(supl): 14-18.

Marino, S., Gallo, J.J., Ford, D.A., & Anthony, J.C. (1995). Filters on the pathway to mental health care. I. Incident mental disorders. *Psychological Medicine*, 25, 1135-1148.

Mason, M.J. (1997). Patterns of service utilization for Mexican American majority students who use alcohol or other drugs. *Journal of Health and Social Policy*, 9(2), 21-28.

Medina-Mora, M.E., Gómez-Mont, F., & Campillo-Serrano C. (1981). Validity and reliability of a high school drug use questionnaire among Mexican students. *Bulletin on Narcotics*, 33(4), 67-76.

Medina-Mora, M.E., Rojas, E., Juárez, F., Berenzon, S., Carreño, S., Galván, J., Villatoro, J., López, E., Olmedo, R., Ortiz, E., & Néquiz, G. (1993). Consumo de sustancias con efectos psicotrópicos en la población estudiantil de enseñanza media y media superior de la República Mexicana [Substance consumption with psychotropic effects in the middle and high school student population of the Republic of Mexico]. *Salud Mental*, 16(3), 2-8.

Medina-Mora, M.E., Berenzon, S., López, E.K., Solís, L., Caballero, M.A., & González, J. (1997). El uso de servicios de salud por los pacientes con trastornos mentales: Resultados de una encuesta en una población de escasos recursos [The use of health services by mentally disturbed patients: Results of a low resource population survey]. *Salud Mental*, 20(supl), 32-38.

Medina-Mora, M.E, Villatoro JA., Fleiz, C. (1999). Estudio de niñas, niños y adolescentes entre 6 y 17 años trabajadores en 100 ciudades. Capítulo de uso indebido de sustancias. [Study of working girls, boys, and adolescents between 6 and 17 in 100 cities. Chapter on illicit drug use]. Mexico: DIF Nacional, UNICEF, PNUFID.

Nelson, B.V., Patience, T.H., & MacDonald, D.C. (1999). Adolescent risk behavior and the influence of parents and education. *Journal of the American Board of Family Practice*, 12(6), 436-443.

Offer, D., Howard, K.I., Schonert, K.A., & Ostrov, E. (1991). To whom do adolescents turn for help? Differences between disturbed and nondisturbed adolescents. *Journal of the American Academy of Child & Adolescent Psychiatry*, 30(4), 623-630.

Ortiz, A., Rodríguez, E., Galván, J., Soriano, A., Flores, J.C. (1999). *Tendencias recientes del uso de drogas. Sistema de Registro de Información en Drogas SRID* [Recent trends in drug use. Drug Information Registry System]. Reporte No. 26. Instituto Mexicano de Psiquiatría. México.

Richardson, J.L., Radziszewska, B., Dent, C.W., & Flay, B.R. (1993). Relationship between after-school care of adolescents and substance use, risk taking, depressed mood, and academic achievement. *Pediatrics*, 92(1), 32-38.

Rojas, E., Medina-Mora, M.E., Villatoro, J., Juárez, F., Carreño, S., & Berenzon, S. (1998). Evolución del consumo de drogas entre estudiantes del Distrito Federal [Evolution of drug consumption in Federal District students]. *Salud Mental*, 21(1), 37-42.

Rosovsky, H., Cravioto, P., & Medina-Mora, M.E. (Comps). (1999). *El Consumo de drogas en México. Diagnóstico. Tendencias. Acciones*. [Drug use in Mexico. Diagnosis. Trends. Actions]. Mexico: Secretaría de Salud/CONADIC.

Solís, L.R., & Medina-Mora, M.E. (1994). La utilización de servicios de atención para la salud mental por mujeres mexicanas. Resultados de dos encuestas Nacionales [The utilization of mental health services by Mexican women: Results of two national surveys]. *Salud Mental*, 17(1), 7-10.

StataCorp. (1999). Stata Statistical Software. Release 6.0. Reference Manual. Texas: Stata Press.

Stronski, S.M., Ireland, M., Michaud, P., Narring, F., & Resnick, M.D. (2000). Protective correlates of stages in adolescent substance use: A Swiss National Study. *Journal of Adolescent Health*, 26(6), 420-427.

Villatoro, J.A., Andrade, P., Fleiz, C., Medina-Mora, M.E., Reyes, I., & Rivera, E. (1997). La relación padres-hijos: Una escala para evaluar el ambiente familiar de los adolescentes [Parent-child relations: A scale for evaluating the family environment of adolescents]. *Salud Mental*, 20(2), 21-27.

Villatoro, J.A., Medina-Mora, M.E., Cardiel, H., Fleiz, C., Alcántar, E., Hernández, S., Parra, J., & Néquiz, G. (1999). La situación del consumo de sustancias entre estudiantes de la ciudad de México. Medición otoño de 1997 [The substance consumption situation in Mexico City students: Autumn 1997 measurement]. *Salud Mental*, 22(2), 18-30.

American Beauty???

Kathy Rabin

Let me ask each of you what comes to mind when you think of American Beauty? For me it could be the graceful coast of California, the beautiful untouched snow, solitude, and silence of Yellowstone National Park in the winter, the lush forests lining the Hudson River or even the Alaskan Glaciers as they tumble powerfully into Glacier Bay. All of this is part of what we could imagine as beautiful in our land of America. Unfortunately, I will not be speaking about our country's physical beauty but rather of a human landscape that is anything but beautiful.

A few weeks ago, with my husband Neil being away on business, Brooke, our 14-year-old and Lauren our 16-year-old and I were looking for a movie to see together I browsed the papers and noticed that the film *American Beauty* was nominated for numerous Academy awards. I thought this must be an excellent movie to have received so many possible accolades. Although it was R rated, I had been comfortable in the past with many R rated movies my girls had seen.

Hoping to enjoy this one as well, we headed to the movie for a special evening together.

Together we were, but I was sorry with the selection of the movie. With Brooke on one side of me and Lauren on the other, I became more uncomfortable and disturbed as the movie progressed. I even contemplated leaving. I decided to stay, but with great trepidation. I realized that as much as I might want to, I cannot shelter them completely from the harsh and ugly aspects of the world we live in today and chose to fin-

[Haworth co-indexing entry note]: "American Beauty???" Rabin, Kathy. Co-published simultaneously in *Journal of Family Social Work* (The Haworth Social Work Practice Press, an imprint of The Haworth Press, Inc.) Vol. 6, No. 1, 2001. pp. 97-99; and: *Families and Health: Cross-Cultural Perspectives* (ed: Jorge Delva) The Haworth Social Work Practice Press, an imprint of The Haworth Press, Inc., 2001, pp.97-99. Single or multiple copies of this article are available for a fee from The Haworth Document Delivery Service [1-800-342-9678, 9:00 a.m. - 5:00 p.m. (EST). E-mail address: getinfo@haworthpressinc.com].

ish the movie, knowing I would make it an opportunity for discussion later over dinner.

Perhaps raising two teenage daughters in today's world heightens my awareness of messages that are taken from movies such as this. Messages that force upon us a sense of what is normal and acceptable and what impressionable young people take in as truth.

It was not long after I saw this movie that I was in a discussion with a few teenagers, where I voiced my objection to this film. One teenager spoke out and said, "But this is the way the world is, this is reality." You can imagine how this statement disturbed me even more; the fact that this teenager did not question what was being depicted, was immune to the deviant themes this film portrayed, and was perceiving the behavior enacted as normal and acceptable.

I assure you that I am not naive to the fact that problems exist in families and that no family lives in a complete utopia. What concerns me is not that problems exist but rather the extreme to which they are depicted and the fact that we seem to have come to unquestionably accept them as normal. Through the movies and videos we watch the words in songs we hear, and the people we have come to idolize. Evil somehow has become okay.

American Beauty is nothing more than dysfunction at its best or should I say its worst. America, unfortunately, maybe has come to this. "Beauty" it is not!

The American landscape described in this movie is not beautiful. It shows the destruction of family, the death of the American dream, it glorifies materialism, infidelity, drug use, guns and violence and accentuates society's obsession with sexuality.

I am disturbed by the constant bombardment of messages forced upon us through movies like this, TV programs, music, and the glut of commercials inundating our lives and, especially, all of those aimed at children and teens. Today more than ever, messages about how one should look, think and act are obvious.

I see children hurried out of their innocence long before they are ready. I believe they are surrounded by excessive portrayals of what someone else considers acceptable reality. While our children need to be educated so that they are able to function in a world that is not always beautiful, certainly this needs to happen gradually with sensitivity and care by the people who know them best.

What are kids doing with the messages contained in what they see and hear? Unless we listen we may not know. Most likely, they view them as acceptable since they lack the critical thinking skills and life experience required to make a sound judgment.

It is time to inspire our youth. We need to expect more and teach more. We must emphasize good values and responsible morals. We must encourage respect and kindness. We must be competent role models. We must show them the beauty of a radiant smile and a tender touch. We must stand up and make our point and question what we see and hear as we see and hear it. We must listen to young people's views and reasoning, and demonstrate critical thinking and effective assessment skills to help them develop theirs.

The time has come to raise the standards. An awareness of what we have become and what could be is a good start. Perhaps we can soon be entertained by what is wholesome and good, what life should and could be and what we might strive towards as people, parents, grandparents and children.

We can turn to our own Jewish heritage, the Ten Commandments, the 613 Mitzvoth from the torah, the lessons we learn from the torah and from our rich history; all can serve as guides toward living a life of true beauty.

Hopefully I have raised your awareness about how vulnerable our children and teenagers are to the uncensored and harsh world in which we live. I pray that those of us here will make a commitment to impact the lives of young people, whether it is our own child, grandchild, niece, nephew or just a friend. We must stop for a moment and make a point that what we hear and see is not good or beautiful and when it is let them know that as well. They must know when we don't approve. They must know to expect more. They must know to question what has become popular and accepted in our culture.

Each one of us can make a difference and paint a landscape of human life that contains beauty and grace just as God our Creator intended. Amen.

AUTHOR NOTE

Kathy Rabin is Vice-President of Congregation Gates of Prayer in Metairie, LA. Reform Jewish tradition encourages a D'Var Torah–Torah teaching–prior to meetings of the Board of Trustees. Kathy chose to share these comments in lieu of a Torah teaching. Inspired by her comments, she was asked by the Congregation Rabbi to share these comments at a Friday evening service as an alternative to his sermon.

Index

Page numbers followed by "f" indicate figures; "t" following a page number indicates tabular material.

For Product Safety Concerns and Information please contact our EU
representative GPSR@taylorandfrancis.com Taylor & Francis Verlag GmbH,
Kaufingerstraße 24, 80331 München, Germany

Batch number: 08158221

Printed by Printforce, the Netherlands